Parental Alienation

This book provides a comprehensive overview of established evidence-based interventions for the problems inherent in parental alienation.

The book focuses on helping families and ensuring the needs of the child are met. Increasing attention has been given to the subject of parental alienation in recent years, as divorce rates have increased and more children are being brought up in the context of ongoing parental conflict, risking significant emotional harm. Chapters point to the application of numerous evidence-based interventions that are already available and detail how to identify, assess and intervene effectively with families where parental alienation has been identified.

This text will be of interest to those working in the family courts, particularly expert witnesses, clinical psychologists, therapists, social workers, guardians and other legal professionals, in addition to researchers with an interest in parental alienation.

Denise McCartan, PhD, DClinPsych, is an HCPC Registered Clinical Psychologist, who also has a research doctorate and has published her work in peer-reviewed journals. She is an Associate Fellow of The British Psychological Society (BPS), Chartered Psychologist and Chartered Scientist. As a Court Expert Witness, she has assessed hundreds of families in the family courts.

Parental Alienation

An Evidence-Based Approach

Denise McCartan

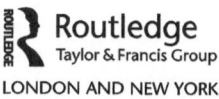
Routledge
Taylor & Francis Group

LONDON AND NEW YORK

First published 2022
by Routledge
4 Park Square, Milton Park, Abingdon, Oxon OX14 4RN

and by Routledge
605 Third Avenue, New York, NY 10158

Routledge is an imprint of the Taylor & Francis Group, an informa business

© 2022 Denise McCartan

British Library Cataloguing-in-Publication Data
A catalogue record for this book is available from the British Library

Library of Congress Cataloging-in-Publication Data
A catalog record for this book has been requested

ISBN: 978-0-367-74115-0 (hbk)
ISBN: 978-0-367-74113-6 (pbk)
ISBN: 978-1-003-15614-7 (ebk)

DOI: 10.4324/9781003156147

Typeset in Times New Roman
by Apex CoVantage, LLC

Contents

Acknowledgements

To: Nadia, Clara and Imogen

Chapter 1

Understanding parental alienation

Introduction – how did this book happen?

In 2010, along with three others, I was invited to speak to a group of around 200 lay magistrates. The other speakers were a consultant psychiatrist, a senior barrister (Queen's Counsel) and a keynote speaker who was a High Court judge. We had been asked to talk about 'Contact' and had prepared our talks independently of each other. I was fairly new to family court work and had read the research around the topic. I was aware that a certain percentage of children did not wish to attend contact and discussed the advantages to maintaining a relationship with both parents. This was not the information the audience needed. The overwhelming issue that attendees wanted to discuss was what to do when it was reported a child did not want to attend contact with a parent who no longer lived with them. The attendees were child-focused and wondered whether any intervention could be considered to try to bring about change. The group presented as concerned about the number of cases that they saw and frustrated with the lack of available options for bringing about change.

At the meeting, the barrister was clearly very familiar with the issues. He acknowledged it was a problem. The psychiatrist, who had worked in the courts for many years, appeared unsurprised and said children 'do not like the dentist' but their parents had to take them. There was clearly a lack of solutions and a lot of questions from the audience, who presented as though they were at a loss with the issues. Unfamiliar with parental alienation at that time, I felt unprepared and was unable to offer any helpful advice.

The event itself was educative and stimulating and highlighted the difficulties that those trying to work with families in the court system were presented with regularly. There were many issues relating to contact between parents after separation, and no intervention had been discussed or developed. As I became more involved in family court work, I reflected on the difficulties and began to see more private family law cases. I was aware that when couples separated and they had children, there were frequently contentious situations whereby allegations and counter-allegations were made; however, I did not know the extent of the problem. Often negative comments about the other person's parenting ability were made, but in the most complex cases, they became more personal and sometimes the resident parent stopped the non-resident parent from seeing the children

DOI: 10.4324/9781003156147-1

altogether. This was often accompanied by a claim that the children did not want to attend contact and would see the non-resident parent when they were older. There were also occasions when the non-resident parent was accused of physical abuse and/or sexual assault. There was little or no evidence associated with the allegations, and the accused parent suggested the claims were associated with malice. Often the other parent had no history that suggested they might present a risk to their child, and the focus appeared to be on stopping the non-resident parent from seeing the child.

Around the same time, in my clinical practice a lot of cases with this presentation were emerging. As there are two perspectives to any relationship breakdown, both parents were usually spoken to when advice was required in relation to a child's welfare and contact issues. Often, the resident parent indicated they thought that the child should discontinue contact with their non-resident parent, and sometimes they exerted pressure on me to agree with this. I noticed that sometimes if one parent rang independently of a court order to make an appointment, saying they needed advice, the consultation did not proceed if I said I would like to speak to both parents. I also became aware that typically in private family law cases, both parents had differing viewpoints about their situation with respect to contact and sometimes there was really very little they agreed on. With increasing frequency, the term 'parental alienation' cropped up, and when I began to look at the extensive literature, I discovered that this term described a group of behaviours that were observed in the court and were very familiar to legal and social services professionals working with private family law practices.

The term 'parental alienation' is often used in child contact disputes, although not in health care settings. This is because although the behaviours can have a significant impact on an individual's social, emotional, behavioural and cognitive functioning, it is the associated outcomes that might require intervention. For example, if the individual involved experienced anxiety and depression or another mental health issue associated with their experiences during a complex relationship separation, they might need therapeutic intervention or support. The behaviours, thoughts and feelings and their impact on emotional wellbeing would be the focus of a mental health assessment. The term 'parental alienation' has gradually moved into mainstream use and is relevant to any mental health assessment because it is likely to indicate high levels of stress for all involved. Despite this there continue to be many publications that dismiss or minimise it. When the behaviours are broken down and considered, it is difficult to deny the situation completely, and most people working in private family law are aware that parental alienation does occur. At the severe end it is extremely stressful for all involved, including professionals trying to help, and it can have long-term implications for the children who are caught in the mix and their parents.

Parental Alienation

The issue of parental alienation (PA) typically arises after parents have separated. The term is used to describe a situation whereby one parent has a negative influence on a child's relationship with the other parent and makes a deliberate effort to intervene and prevent the relationship from developing/continuing or improving. These behaviours are often associated with deterioration or termination of the relationship, or in some cases, if the parents' relationship ends before the child begins to put down memories, it never really begins, e.g. if the non-resident parent leaves home before a baby is born. PA is a problem that is relevant to and has a significant negative impact on many families. The issue straddles psychology, law and sociology, and it has been noted that the association with more than one discipline leads to professionals writing about concepts that they encounter but that are not directly within their area (1). It could be argued that PA represents a range of difficulties that are relevant to all three disciplines, depending on which aspect is examined. Over time it appears that a consensus about what constitutes PA is slowly emerging. There is an interest in understanding the concept and attempting to address the difficulties that cause significant harm and distress to many families.

PA is therefore a form of manipulation, and usually one parent influences a child or children so that they view the other parent negatively. It typically occurs after the relationship between the parents has ended, although it may begin when both parents live at home. The manipulation results in deterioration or complete cessation of the relationship between the 'targeted' parent and the child. The 'targeted' parent is often one with whom the child previously had a positive relationship and is usually the non-resident parent, whilst the 'alienating' parent is typically the resident parent and therefore has more opportunity to influence their child to believe that the targeted parent is not someone they want to have a relationship with or continue to view positively.

The difficulties have been traced back to a court case describing PA 215 years ago (1). Since that time many psychiatrists and behavioural scientists have referred to the issues associated with a child rejecting a parent for no apparent reason, although the rejection appears to be associated with the behaviour of the other parent (1). The term 'brainwashed' was introduced to this discussion to explain why often the child presented as having practised assertions that sounded similar to the alienating parent's statements, and they tended to hold firm a view that mirrored that of the resident parent.

The term 'parental alienation' is often described as the development of the child psychiatrist Richard Gardner's (1970) reflections that children of divorced couples often aligned themselves with one parent and refused to see the other one. Gardner wrote extensively about this issue and is generally recognised as one of the first people to draw attention to the frequency with which this occurs. Typically, the child also refused to see the targeted parent's extended family. Today couples do not necessarily marry and divorce, and many children are born from parents who do not remain in a relationship. When couples separate, children often live with one parent, who is known as the 'resident parent', and have periods of contact with the 'non-resident parent', although there are a number of different models of parenting used after separation, such as co-parenting (the parents are amicable and share care of their child) and parallel parenting (the parents do not communicate, but the child sees both parents). Some couples manage to share care of their children amicably; however, many non-resident parents do not have an opportunity to bond with their child in the same manner as the resident parent, particularly if the couple separates before the child is born. Nevertheless, many non-resident parents would like to continue or begin to have a relationship with their child, and there are of course significant benefits for the child if this can be managed appropriately.

A word about language

Language can be emotive, and this is particularly the case in contentious private family law cases. Terms like 'targeted parent' suggest there is a victim, and others like 'alienating parent' could suggest intention or be perceived as blaming. Also, there are occasions when the targeted parent becomes the alienating parent and vice versa, which could make any discussion about the situation confusing. Nevertheless, to make this text congruent with some others, I am using the terms 'alienating' and 'targeted' parents, and I hope the reader will understand that I am neither attributing blame nor suggesting victimhood (2). The victims in contentious contact cases are the children, and most professionals do not lose sight of that.

In my experience those who wish to criticise the concept of PA manipulate the weaknesses in the data gathered so far, and they use language from previous negative publications to support their arguments. Before and during the writing of this book, I read many peer-reviewed papers about PA, and I was taken aback by how often authors wrote misleading information. For example, one academic publication reported that in one particular, private family law case, after the children were placed in the care of their father, they never saw their mother again. I emailed the writer and asked for further information, and I was kindly sent the judgement, which had been published. The writer indicated the relevant paragraphs that I should read. When I read them, the judge had said the father was not to prevent the children from seeing their mother. There were no indications that this had actually happened. There was no reference to any follow-up on the case, to check whether the children saw the mother again. I asked some colleagues to read the judgment in case I misinterpreted it, and it seemed impossible to extract the writer's understanding from the information published. In a similar misunderstanding of language, and in another peer-reviewed paper, I read that a child had been 'handcuffed' and brought to a 'reunification camp' (an intervention to help the child reunite with their 'alienated' parent). I contacted someone associated with the camp and was told the child was 17 years old and, when travelling through an airport, said they had a bomb, so airport security handcuffed them. Therefore, when writing this book, it seemed impossible at times to write about the seemingly contentious concept of PA without checking every single detail.

In writing this book I wanted to identify the current status of PA in the context of the literature, both positive and negative, and consider how this applies in the UK. That proved to be a little more tricky than anticipated, as many authors have written negatively about PA and then gone on to describe their version of it, which is different from mainstream use of the term. This makes for a lively debate when authors are arguing about different concepts or misinterpreting/misrepresenting the writings of others, although it made it difficult to write about PA. The goal of this book is to try to understand the seemingly confusing and unwieldy situation that occurs in private family law and can have a devastating impact on families and, more importantly, to think about possible interventions and approaches to remediation or resolution.

The history

As already noted, the term 'parental alienation' is believed to have initially been coined in the 1970's by Richard Gardner (3), a psychiatrist who worked with children and families. Gardner also completed assessments and wrote reports for the courts as an expert witness. Gardner raised the profile of this issue, wrote about it and proposed 'parental alienation syndrome' (PAS), which he felt should be included as a psychiatric disorder in the *Diagnostic and Statistical Manual* (*DSM*) (a manual describing disorders, used by health care providers for diagnosis). As Gardner was medically trained it seems reasonable that he would apply a medical model approach to the issues, and this is likely to explain his reasoning for suggesting that the problems constituted a 'syndrome'.

Although Gardner had his critics, PAS was at one stage proposed for entry to the *DSM*. The following criteria was proposed for PAS (4):

1   A campaign of denigration towards the 'targeted' parent.
2   Weak, absurd or frivolous rationalisations for the deprecation.
3   A lack of ambivalence about the situation.
4   The 'independent-thinker' phenomenon – the child reports that their thoughts about the 'targeted' parent are independent of the 'alienating' parent's influence.
5   Unquestioning support of the alienating parent in the parental conflict.
6   Absence of guilt over cruelty to and/or exploitation of the targeted parent.
7   The presence of borrowed scenarios, for example, the targeted parent 'dropped me on my head when I was a baby'.
8   Spread of the animosity to the friends and/or extended family of the targeted parent.

It was argued that a lack of awareness of PAS explained its absence from the *DSM*, and Gardner called on professionals and the public to contact the *DSM* editors and tell them about their experiences of parental alienation (5). It was noted that critics of the concept had submitted information to *DSM* that might be influential in ensuring PAS was not recognised as a 'disorder'. Gardner was quite a lone voice at times, trying to raise the profile of this difficulty, and others commented that Gardner's greatest insight was to recognise that not all allegations made against a parent during parental separation are true (6). Since Gardner's time, the arguments have continued about whether PAS could be appropriately used as a diagnosis. Some have moved away from the idea of a diagnosis towards use of the term 'parental alienation' in the way the term 'domestic violence' is used, and in that way, it is accepted as a group of behaviours.

This is helpful as it means everyone understands what the term refers to, without the emotional loading attached to a diagnosis (although some diagnoses are relevant to or result from PA). Most people working in the family courts are now familiar with the term, and it is increasingly recognised as appropriate and valid. However, numerous difficulties remain; for example, the harm caused by PA can be difficult to prove and quantify, and it is an issue for professional assessment to ensure that the problems are not attributed to PA when there are other explanations for the behaviours (7).

At the same time as Gardner wrote about his observations, a social worker called Leona Kopetski, without knowledge of his work, was collecting data for the Child and Family Evaluation Team in Colorado, and after considering the information gathered from 413 families involved in residency disputes, her team reached similar conclusions to those of Gardner, although there were also some differences (8). It was noted that parental alienation (syndrome) was a form of 'psycho-social pathology' that resulted from an alienating parent having difficulty adjusting to their situation, in the context of ambivalence, narcissistic injury (the alienating parent reacts poorly to criticism), internal conflict or threats to their self-esteem (8). Alienating parents tended to align themselves with proven theories or causes and to accuse the targeted parent of not behaving appropriately. It was reported that alienating parents often believed the allegations that they made against the targeted parent, and the following process was described (8):

1   The alienating parent holds a negative view of the targeted parent, of which the child is aware. Over time the child comes to hold the same view as the alienating parent.
2   The alienating parent claims the child is distressed both before and after contact with the targeted parent. The targeted parent does not observe this during contact. As soon as the child is old enough to give an opinion, they refuse to see the targeted parent.
3   The alienating parent exhibits fear, anger and 'protectiveness' towards the child. The child presents similarly. Solutions are either rejected or attempted and sabotaged.
4   There is some discussion about the 'trauma' the child will experience if they are separated from their 'primary attachment figure'. There is sometimes a reference to the 'child's right to be heard', e.g. 'they don't want to go'.
5   The alienating parent often talks about 'justice' and their right to be heard. They appear to view their contact with the child as a 'reward' and the targeted parent's alienation as a 'punishment'.
6   The need of the child to have a relationship with both parents is not considered. In the alienating parent's view, the child will have a relationship with only one parent: either them or the targeted parent.

It was also noted that the alienating parent's expressed fear was that the court expert would not see the pathology in the targeted parent. Anyone who challenged the alienating parent could be accused of being naïve, charmed or brainwashed by the targeted parent. They might also be accused of being biased towards them or incompetent. Assessors who held a view opposing the alienating parent were also often accused of collaborating with the targeted parent to harm the child (8).

It was also noted that a 'normal' parent making an allegation was aware that flaws are part of the human condition and was relieved when concerns were unfounded; however, alienating parents were angry and disappointed when it was found that their child had not been hurt. In addition, 'normal' parents understood that their child would have positive relationships with others and continued to feel some affection for the ex-partner. It was concluded that PA worked by exploiting the usual concerns that professionals have when dealing with complex family cases (8).

Over time, there have been a number of publications about the concept of parental alienation and whether or not it constitutes a syndrome, and many authors have argued about this issue. The *Diagnostic and Statistical Manual*'s fifth edition (*DSM*-V) (9) made reference to some of the behaviours observed in parental alienation, under the diagnostic code V995.51, 'Child Psychological Abuse'. In relation to parental alienation, the behaviours refer to a situation whereby a parent or caregiver may berate, humiliate or threaten the child or indicate that another person will harm them or things they care about (10).

Another potentially relevant diagnosis described in the *DSM*-V is V61.29, 'Child Affected by Parental Relationship Distress', which is associated with a situation when the negative influence of the parental relationship conflict has a significant impact on the child's emotional welfare or other medical disorders.

The World Health Organisation's International Classification of Diseases and Related Health Problems, version 11 (ICD-11) (11), is an epidemiological tool, designed to record and analyse conditions that impact on health. It is also used by health care workers for diagnosis. ICD-11 does not recognise PA, but some of the associated problems are referred to in the category QE52.0: Caregiver Child Relationship Problem, which relates to a poor long-term relationship between the caregiver and their child and results in disturbance in functioning. Of course, many alienating parents would say that they have a very positive relationship with their child.

In thinking about whether a diagnosis is helpful, it seems that this is only likely if it leads to a focus on interventions and provides a pathway for professionals to try to improve a child's situation. Many adults and children have been harmed by alienating behaviours, which can result in significant mental health problems, and it could be argued that there has been a preoccupation with the use of terminology. There is, however, also a lack of knowledge about interventions for people who struggle with the issue of contact in contentious family law cases and how to address the problems, which is after all much more important than what the situation is called. Over time there has been an increased acceptance of the term 'parental alienation' by many individuals. It is a concept which most people understand, and the word 'syndrome' is not used. PA has come to be understood as a series of behaviours carried out by the alienating parent in order to disrupt the relationship with the targeted parent. It has been described as a form of domestic violence, and it is increasingly recognised as a problem that impacts on many aspects of a child's functioning (12).

There is now significant research about PA, although of course more needs to be done. Some theories have been developed and hypotheses tested, data has been collected and analysed, and there have been attempts to integrate the data with existing theories. Some of the research has used convenience samples with retrospective information gathered from adults who felt they had been alienated as children or adults who self-identified as targeted parents. There is a crossover between some aspects of PA and the existing body of knowledge about many other aspects of psychological functioning. In addition, there has been a move to refine and define the concept and gain acceptance of the phenomenon by using more rigorous and transparent research. It seems that it is time to support those who are attempting to integrate science with real-life problems.

If we accept the concept of PA and we know how it is defined, then it is necessary to consider how and where it presents, how it is assessed and whether it is harmful to children and adults involved. If so, what harm occurs, and which interventions need to be put in place to prevent or ameliorate this? We also need to consider how outcomes are to be measured, i.e. what does success look like? The controversy surrounding the use of the term 'parental alienation' causes anxiety to professionals involved, and there is concern around adopting it. At the same time, it is obvious to most people working in the courts that this situation arises. Anxiety lies around using the term appropriately and appearing to validate something which has not always been accepted as a valid and reliable construct. It appears that there are now obvious situations whereby parents are trying to prevent their child having contact with their ex-partner, and when the ex-partner uses the term 'parental alienation', the alienating parent claims that the ex-partner or targeted parent is trying to hurt them. Likewise, there may be many situations whereby someone is referring to PA, when in fact there are other reasons for the presentation, which is why appropriate assessment is essential for these complex cases.

The parental alienation process

PA behaviours do not take place on a single occasion but rather involve a process whereby a parent gradually, explicitly and/or implicitly, erodes the absent parent's relationship with their children (13). Children are typically alienated over a period of time by rejection, shame, ridicule or being made to feel guilty if they show any loyalty or warmth to the absent parent or carer. Very often, this process includes the extended family of the targeted parent. The alienating parent is openly or privately hostile, describes the targeted parent negatively and/or may withdraw love or affection when the child shows any signs of thinking positively about the targeted parent. The alienating parent may also share adult information with the children, for example, relating to financial or court matters. Alienation can be carried out very discreetly, and professionals who are not experienced in this field can be easily misled. Also, the velocity of the alienating parent's assertions can be overwhelming for professionals, and they may be charmed by the alienating parent and/or threatened or convinced that the targeted parent presents a risk to the children. There are so many ways that an alienating parent can disrupt the relationship between the child and the targeted parent, and sometimes all of these approaches are used in what results in a battle between the parents that continues for years, sometimes until the child has grown up.

Categories – mild/moderate/severe

It has been suggested that alienating behaviours should be categorised as mild, moderate or severe, and these are described more fully later in this book (6, 14–16). Mild alienating behaviours may occur when parents are going through a difficult time in their relationship or a separation, and one parent complains about the other; however, the criticism is not consistent, and the child is not overly influenced by it (17). When the child is with the targeted parent, they present as comfortable, and alienating parents may later regret this behaviour when they adjust to the separation.

Moderate alienating behaviours involve struggles around contact and parental intervention to attempt to prevent the child having contact with their targeted parent. The child understands that one parent does not like the other and may resist contact, but once with the targeted parent, their behaviour may change over time to become more relaxed so they enjoy their experiences together. Often, the alienating parent does not recognise that they are behaving inappropriately. There is a general consensus that without intervention at this stage, alienating behaviours will continue until the child is in the severe category (7).

The severely alienated child displays many of the issues described by Gardner. They typically express strong views about the targeted parent. They may say they are frightened of them or accuse them of abandoning or not loving them; they say they do not like them; they are not good people. If attempts are made to try to introduce indirect contact (in my experience this tends to involve sending cards or gifts through solicitors), the child will say the targeted parent bought them the wrong gifts and reject them, and cards may be destroyed. The child will sometimes say that if they are made to see their targeted parent, they will hide, run away, etc. Sometimes the alienating parent says that if the targeted parent would 'leave them alone', then the child may have contact with them at some stage in the future. In more extreme cases, children self-harm and/or threaten to 'kill' themselves or the target parent for 'ruining their lives' by taking the alienating parent to court. They may experience significant mental health problems. Attempts by professionals to try to engage the child with the targeted parent result in rejection of the targeted parent and sometimes quite a lot of verbal abuse and name-calling of everyone involved by the child, except the alienating parent. At the same time the alienating parent often maintains a stance that they want the child to see the targeted parent and are not involved in the child's assertions.

It has been reported that a moderately or severely alienated child will present with the following (7):

- The behaviour will be chronic, although can be intermittent.
- The behaviour is frequent.
- The behaviour is present in most situations.
- It occurs without any demonstrations of fondness towards the targeted parent.
- The behaviour is towards only the targeted parent and not the alienating parent.
- The behaviour is unusual for the child's developmental stage.
- It appears that the behaviour is not in keeping with the history of the targeted parent's presentation.

When parental alienation is misidentified

There are occasions when PA is identified when it is not present, and professionals have misunderstood the concept or the situation. Attempts to address the nuances of this situation point out that not all negative behaviours towards a parent indicate that the child has been alienated (7, 18). Most professional people appreciate this fact and do not jump to conclusions, but rather try to understand the reasons for the child's behaviour. There are many different situations when a child may not wish to have contact with a non-resident parent; for example, the child may have a temperament that is difficult to manage, or if they are teenagers, they may be difficult on one occasion (this second situation is unlikely to reach court). Other potential situations when a child may not wish to see their non-resident parent are if the child is anxious about leaving the resident parent because they are concerned about them, or they do not like the non-resident parent's partner or a member of their extended family or a friend, or the child does not feel comfortable in the non-resident parent's home and misses spending time with their friends in their locality. As will be discussed, it is entirely possible that the child is naturally more aligned with one parent than with the other (see Chapter 4 for further discussion around this) (7). Also, as children approach their teenage years, they are beginning to align with their friends rather than their parents, and they may naturally feel they want to spend less time with both of their parents.

The term 'parental alienation' can be misused, and when this occurs, it undermines the validity of PA and adds to the scepticism that some feel about the concept. For that reason, some advise thorough investigation by professionals to ensure that PA is not raised as an issue when it is not present and to explore whether there may be other possible explanations for behaviour (7).

Justified estrangement or rejection

If the child has been exposed to domestic violence by the non-resident parent when they lived at the family home, then they may not wish to continue to have a relationship with them after they leave. Or if the non-resident parent has mistreated the child in the past, this is likely to make it difficult for the child to engage with them. They may be frightened of the parent, and a threat may be present, even if the parent states they have changed their behaviour. The child may be relieved that they no longer have to live with the non-resident parent and hope they do not have to see them again.

In addition, if a child attends contact and the non-resident parent does not fully engage with them but expects the child to be happy to see them simply because they are a parent, the contact is unlikely to be sustainable. Some parents believe it is sufficient to collect their child and either take them to, or drop them off at, a grandparent's or extended family member's home, without engaging with the child. In my experience, this is okay sometimes, if the child has a good relationship with the grandparents or extended family, but if the non-resident parent rarely spends time with a child, then the child can feel rejected, and even if they enjoy seeing other relatives sometimes, they may eventually give up on the likelihood of spending time with their non-resident parent. At the same time the non-resident parent is missing an opportunity to develop their relationship with their child. I have also observed contacts where parents spend a lot of time looking at their mobile phones, or they are simply out of sync with the child and speak to them as if they were at a different developmental stage, and it is easy to see how a child might be reluctant to attend contact in this situation. The issues of justified estrangement are discussed more fully in Chapter 4.

Hybrids

'Enmeshment' is a term used to describe a situation whereby two individuals become so entangled in the other's emotional state that the boundaries become blurred, so, for example, usually if one is happy, the other is happy. It has been noted that a child rarely refuses contact for one particular reason, and they may refuse contact because of a combination of factors that include enmeshment, estrangement and alienation. This is referred to as a 'hybrid' situation. Hybrid cases can include both rational and irrational reasoning for declining contact with the targeted parent. For example, most children can find a reason to criticise their parents; however, if they are supported by an alienating parent to do this, it makes relationship recovery more challenging for the targeted parent (7). This means that if an assessment is required for court purposes, it is essential that it is carried out by an appropriate evaluator who understands the nuances of PA behaviours and can identify a hybrid if required. Hybrid presentations are discussed more fully in Chapter 4.

Conclusion

PA and associated difficulties present significant issues for those working in the family courts. PA occurs when a resident parent manipulates a child to try to undermine the child's relationship with a non-resident parent. Many independent court experts from different parts of the world have recognised the problems and attempted to describe these in the literature. Although there have been disparities in their accounts of the observed behaviours and their consequences, there have also been many similarities, leading to an increasing acceptance of the terminology. There is now a consensus about what PA is and the negative impact it has on children and families.

Some authors have moved away from the argument about whether PA is a valid concept and have accepted the terminology for the purposes of their investigation and writing (2, 7, 19). There is general acceptance of the concept, and this appears to result from knowledge derived through a combination of clinical experience in the context of the literature. Most people seem to agree that more research is needed. The literature is evolving at present, and there are many academics and clinicians trying to define and refine the concept of PA so that it can be used as a valid and reliable construct and aid outcomes for these complicated cases.

The concerns of those who work with this complex group often relate to: How precisely does it happen, and can it be prevented? Why does someone alienate their child from the other parent? If it is understood, then it increases the likelihood of finding an intervention. The most important outcomes relate to whether there are adverse effects on any child involved, and if so, what are they? What can be done to try to reduce or ameliorate the impact of these behaviours on children? Those who try to address the issue do so sometimes in opposition to alienating parents, which makes the work both challenging and overwhelming at times.

The situation is more complex than understood by many, which is why professionals need education about PA and good personal and professional support networks. Over time, the notion of parental alienation as a concept has been discussed and criticised; however, the term has survived. No matter what it is called, how it is referred to or whether some professionals like or dislike the term, there are occasions when one parent influences their child so that they withdraw from the relationship with the absent parent. This process is increasingly referred to as 'parental alienation'.

References

1   Lorandos, D. (2020). Parental alienation in U.S. Courts, 1985 to 2018. *Family Court Review*, 58, 322–339.
2   Haines, J., Matthewson, M. and Turnbull, M. (2020). *Understanding and managing parental alienation: A guide to assessment and intervention*. Oxon: Routledge.
3   Gardner, R.A. (1970). *The boys and girls book about divorce*. New York, NY: Penguin Random House.
4   Gardner, R.A. (1998). *The parental alienation syndrome* (2nd edition). Cresskill, NJ: Creative Therapeutics, Inc.
5   Gardner, R.A. (2002). *PAS and the DSM-V: A call for action*. Mensdaily.com.
6   Rand, D.C. (1997). The spectrum of parental alienation syndrome (part I). *The American Journal of Forensic Psychology*, 15, 1–50. www.sakkyndig.com/psykologi/artvit/rand1996.pdf.

7   Warshak, R.A. (2019). When evaluators get it wrong: False positive IDs and parental alienation. *Psychology, Public Policy and Law*, 26, 54–68. doi:10.1037/law0000216.

8   Kopetski, L. (1998). Identifying cases of parental alienation syndrome – part 1. *The Colorado Lawyer*, 27, 65–68.

9   American Psychiatric Association. (2013). *Diagnostic and statistical manual of mental disorders: DSM-5*. Arlington, VA: American Psychiatric Association.

10 Von Boch-Galhau, W. (2018). Parental alienation (syndrome) – A serious form of psychological child abuse. *Mental Health and Family Medicine*, 14, 725–739.

11 World Health Organisation. (2018). *International classification of diseases for mortality and morbidity statistics* (11th edition). https://icd.who.int/browse11/l-m/en.

12 Harman, J.J., Kruk, E. and Hines, D.A. (2018). Parental alienating behaviors: An unacknowledged form of family violence. *Psychological Bulletin*, 144, 1275–1299. doi:10.1037/bu10000175.

13 Verrocchio, M.C., Baker, A.J.K. and Marchett, D. (2017). Adult report of childhood exposure to parent alienation at different developmental time periods. *Journal of Family Therapy*, 40, 602–618. doi:10.1111/1467-6427.12192.

14 Gardner, R.A., Sauber, R.S. and Lorandos, D. (Eds.). (2006). *The international handbook of parental alienation syndrome: Conceptual, clinical and legal considerations*. Springfield, IL: Charles C. Thomas Publisher.

15 Warshak, R.A. (2013). *Severe cases of parental alienation*. In D. Lorandos, W. Bernet and S.R. Sauber (Eds.), *American series in behavioral science and law. Parental alienation: The handbook for mental health and legal professionals* (pp. 125–162). Springfield, IL: Charles C. Thomas Publisher.

16 Sîrbu, A.G., Vintila, M., Tisu, L., Stefanut, A.M., Tudorel, O.I., Maguran, B. and Toma, R.A. (2021). Parental alienation – development and validation of a behavioral anchor scale. *Sustainability*. doi:10.3390/su13010316.

17 Cummings, E.M. and Davies, P.T. (2010). *Marital conflict and children: An emotional security perspective*. New York: Guilford Press.

18 Friedlander, S. and Walters, M.G. (2010). When a child rejects a parent: Tailoring the intervention to fit the problem. *Family Court Review*, 48, 98–111. doi:10/1111/j.1744-1617.2009.01291.x.

19 Harman, J.J., Bernet, W. and Harman, J. (2019). Parental alienation: The blossoming of a field of study. *Current Directions in Psychological Science*, 28, 212–217. doi:10.1177/0963721419827271.

Chapter 2

Why is it important, and what does it look like?

Introduction

As discussed in Chapter 1, parental alienation is a situation that typically occurs during parental separation, whereby one parent, usually the primary caregiver, interferes with a child's relationship with their other parent. Sometimes this results in the child no longer having a relationship with their other, 'targeted' parent. There are occasions when it is stated that the child simply does not want contact with the targeted parent, and depending on the level of alienation, the alienating parent can introduce the notion of risk associated with contact. This can leave professionals feeling unsure about whether to encourage the child to spend time with the targeted parent or not. Risks identified or described sometimes include concerns about physical or sexual assault and can present a quandary for any court expert who does not want to place a child in a position where they may be harmed but equally does not want to ignore the possibility that the allegations may be true.

As we said in Chapter 1, PA is a process and usually occurs over time, and it is important for professionals to be aware that it can happen; otherwise they can easily be misled into thinking that contact between a child and a targeted parent is causing harm, and they might support the alienating parent to bring about an end to the child's relationship with their other parent. Education for professionals is key to ensuring PA identification and intervention, if possible.

Is a scientific approach required?

Although the term 'parental alienation' has been around for a long time, it has only recently moved towards mainstream use. Most people working in the family courts, i.e. legal and social work professionals, will understand what is meant when the term is used. PA is increasingly recognised as an issue for some complex family cases. Efforts to apply scientific principles to PA research have been made, and although the research is already significant, it is still in its infancy. Some researchers describe this as a 'blossoming' of PA research (1). Over time the efforts being made to develop this concept into a more robust construct should enable professionals to speak confidently about PA without fear of criticism for

DOI: 10.4324/9781003156147-2

using a controversial term. Despite the controversy, the one thing that most people who write about PA agree on is that more research is needed (2).

Why is parental alienation important?

There is a growing recognition that PA is an issue that is likely to continue to present as a problem in the family courts (1, 3–4). The family structure has changed over the years, and as it evolves, more parents are deciding not to marry. Those who do get involved as a couple may later become separated, divorced, unpartnered or re-partnered. Sometimes this involves children, and so decisions have to be made about where and how to live. Co-parenting is a significant issue for families, and the question of how best to offer a child a safe and optimum experience is of vital importance. It is therefore critical to consider what aspects of parental functioning contribute to a good outcome for children and which issues create problems. In the context of family development, there is an increasing need to recognise the difficulties that children experience when parents do not support each other appropriately and try to introduce accessible interventions to ameliorate any associated damage.

Children have a legal right to see both parents even after they have separated, and this entitlement can be protected by the law. The benefits of having access to both parents are discussed further in the following chapters, and children need to be able to have a loving, conflict-free relationship with their non-resident parent without interference from their resident parent. A scientific approach to PA is necessary to ensure that an evidence-based strategy to the care of children who end up in the legal system as a result of parental conflict can be implemented. Evidence can inform practice, and professionals can be made aware of the best way of evaluating, intervening in and maintaining families who experience the difficulties described in this book.

Families in the UK

According to the Office for National Statistics, during 2019 there were 2.9 million lone-parent families in the UK, which was 14.9% of the families counted (5). Lone-parent mothers represented 86% of the parent type, although lone-parent fathers had grown by 22% during the previous ten years, and the percentage had grown faster than for lone mothers. Same-sex couples were the fastest-growing family group and had grown by 40% during the previous four years. The number of lone parents with dependent children was significantly lower than previous years, and it was thought this may be because there were fewer teenage pregnancies, the number of births was declining, parents may be re-partnering and more women had been postponing childbirth. It was recognised that some of the lone families may result from a situation whereby a partner had died, or a parent might be uncontactable or uninterested in parenting. It was also noted a parent may have chosen to raise their children alone, although there was no further explanation about this. These statistics reflect how the family has changed in recent years as it continues to develop and evolve. Although there do not appear to be any studies to indicate the number of families in the UK who have PA as an issue, it is important that processes are put in place to ensure that families involved can access intervention if needed to support a child to see their non-resident parent, if appropriate.

Prevalence of alienated families

It appears that the prevalence of alienated families has not been collected or published in the UK. In relation to the US and Canada, there have been some studies to consider the prevalence of adults who had been subject to parental alienating behaviours (6). It was recognised that one of the main limitations of the investigations were that not all children exposed to alienating behaviours became alienated. Using an online survey with a series of questions, 1200 individuals were approached by phone and asked whether they had heard of parental alienating behaviours, and the nature of PA was described to them. The investigators went on to ask for more detail about the nature of any alienation identified, and the number of individuals involved was recorded. Around one-third of Canadian responders (35.2%) and almost half of those from the US (48.5%) were separated parents. They were asked to share their experiences, and individuals were required to indicate whether they felt that efforts had been made by an ex-partner to try to change their relationship with their child. The researchers concluded that the prevalence of parents who felt attempts had been made to alienate then from their child was 35.5% in the US and 32% in Canada. Of this group, around 60% felt alienating behaviours had been successful in ending a relationship with one or more of their children. They found that the more severe the alienating behaviours were, the greater the impact on the targeted parent's relationship with their child.

One of the surveys carried out found almost 40% of US parents and more than 50% of Canadian parents indicated they had engaged in PA behaviours at one stage (1). They did not all describe their reasons for this behaviour, although issues raised by the alienating parent related to drug use, emotional instability and physical abuse, and some concluded they did not know why they had engaged in these behaviours. A smaller number said the other parent was 'just bad', they did not like them or they had financial reasons for restricting access.

In another consideration of prevalence of PA in the US by a different research group, 50 college students were interviewed, and it was found 29% of children from divorced homes were at some level alienated from a parent, although not all children who had experienced alienating behaviours were completely alienated (7). It was concluded that although there was a strong link between alienating behaviours and alienation, there were many factors at play when a child became alienated from a parent. Similarly, another study in the US interviewed 118 adult children of divorce, and it was found that 59.5% reported exposure to alienating behaviours (8). Overall, based on the studies that have been carried out, it seems that around one-third of children from separated families have experienced PA, and a higher percentage were exposed to alienating behaviours. The studies are broadly in keeping with each other and suggest that the behaviours are similar in different regions.

Risk factors for parental alienation

Given that parental separation is on the increase (although lone parenting is not), there is a need to recognise when one parent manipulates their children to ensure they no longer have contact with the absent parent. The child's need to have a relationship with both parents needs to be met and protected.

Identified risk factors for PA would highlight the areas for intervention early on in the process. Risk factors for the emergence of alienation appear to be:

- Sometimes but not always a contentious separation or divorce involving children.
- A resident parent who presents as needing to be in control and will allow contact sometimes in some conditions, typically if it is convenient for them.
- A resident or alienating parent meeting a new partner.
- A non-resident or targeted parent meeting a new partner.

Alienating behaviours used by parents

An alienating parent is one who manipulates their child so they say they do not want contact with their other, targeted parent. A number of behaviours are recognised that indicate PA (9–10). Some of these are discreet, and others are more overt. Some authors described the behaviours as child abuse, noting these would fall beneath the headings of 'emotional/psychological aggression', 'child neglect', 'legal and administrative aggression' and 'physical and sexual aggression' (10).

Emotional/psychological aggression

Emotional/psychological aggression can be characterised by verbal and nonverbal communication with the intention to cause harm. It includes rejecting, deliberately frightening or isolating a child; negatively impacting on a child's thinking; exploiting and/or withholding comfort. It is noted that although they cause significant harm, these behaviours can be difficult to identify and can be carried out covertly so that the behaviours and their impact are not observed by others. Children may also be frightened when a parent criticises the absent parent by creating a belief that the other parent is too dangerous to be around or presents a threat to their integrity. It has been reported that alienating parents regularly invoke anxiety in their child with respect to the targeted parent by reminding them about their safety when they are with them (11). Whilst it is not unusual for a parent to remind their child about the dangers involved with speaking to strangers, an alienating parent can introduce or cultivate fears in a child relating to the other parent's behaviour, resulting in the child feeling the targeted parent is not safe to be around or will not care for them as well as the alienating parent does.

Parents sometimes 'help' children remember events that did not actually occur, or they may exaggerate or embellish memories. This 'memory' may involve harm to the child, the alienating parent and/or another family member, for example a sibling. On many occasions a child has repeated harrowing events that they say happened to either them or their alienating parent when they were a baby. These events typically involve the targeted parent behaving aggressively and are used as explanations as to why the child does not want to attend contact.

On other occasions alienating parents may claim that the targeted parent did not turn up to see their child at, for example, a school production or sports day, when the targeted parent was prevented from knowing about it. They might say the targeted parent has not collected the child when no arrangement had been made. This enables the alienating parent to tell their child that their targeted parent has forgotten about them and diminishes the relationship between the targeted parent and their child. It causes the child emotional distress, which the alienating parent can claim was a result of the targeted parent's behaviour.

During the process, alienating parents also sometimes use children to gather information from the targeted parent on their own behalf. In my experience this typically happens with adolescents, who are old enough to remember to collect the data and skilled enough to access it. In some cases, children tell the alienating parent about text messages or calls that the targeted parent received when they were in their care. Alienating parents then deny that they asked the child to collect this information, saying that the targeted parent left things lying around for the child to see. There may be claims the child saw inappropriate material on a device. This supports the alienating parent's case that the child is not safe in the care of the targeted parent.

A child can be manipulated by rejection, shame or guilt for showing loyalty towards the targeted parent or their family/friends. They can be ridiculed or criticised for appearing to show any positivity towards the targeted parent. The punishment can also involve withdrawal, such as withholding love, affection or comfort if the child does not reject the targeted parent. Sometimes children behave one way towards a targeted parent in the presence of an alienating parent and differently when they are not around.

Another method sometimes used by alienating parents to control a child's behaviour with the targeted parent involves rewarding them for inappropriate behaviour, so if they perform poorly when they meet with the targeted parent or in the presence of professionals, they are given the love, attention, gift, extra time on their device, etc., that they want from the alienating parent. Sometimes when contact time arrives, a child is offered a 'better' alternative with the alienating parent, such as money or a gift or an interesting trip, to try to dissuade them from attending contact.

There are occasions when the child may call the alienating parent by their first name and are aligned with them as a friend. In other cases, the child calls the targeted parent by their first name or tries to change their surname to avoid association with them. In the UK children cannot change their surnames without the support of the alienating parent, although it is typically claimed that this was the child's request.

Alienating parents may interfere with any communication the child has with the targeted parent by insisting on listening to calls from the targeted parent, and they may cut the call short if they desire to do so. In doing so they are modelling rude behaviour to their child. They may claim the conversation was inappropriate. They may read text messages on their child's mobiles or monitor conversations on their devices. Also, in relation to communication, alienating parents may contact the child frequently when they are with the targeted parent, and this can interfere with the quality of contact, particularly if the alienating parent reports they feel unwell or is involved in what is perceived as a more desirable activity. This can result in the child feeling they are either needed at home or missing out on a treat by not being with their other parent.

It has been reported that alienating parents sometimes threaten to harm the targeted parent or their extended family or new partners if they do not behave in a particular way, or they promise rewards for changing behaviours; for example, they say the targeted parent can have contact if they withdraw court applications, although if a court application is withdrawn, the alienating parent does not behave as promised (12). Many targeted parents do not trust the alienating parent enough to proceed with this type of request.

In many cases targeted parents feel threatened by the alienating parent, or they want to protect their child from conflict, and so they avoid meeting them and arrange for the child to be collected by another adult. Sometimes the alienating parent involves another individual, such as a family member, new partner or other adult, to intimidate the targeted parent, and having a third party collect the children can ameliorate this. Sometimes involving a neutral party works, but there are occasions when the alienating parent will not agree to another adult collecting the children and appears to want the opportunity to disparage the targeted parent. Often the presence of the child does not reduce the likelihood of this behaviour. In many cases parents record the 'pick-up' or 'drop-off' on their mobile phones, so that they have 'evidence' of any poor behaviour on the part of the alienating parent during collection for contact or at return time. Some targeted parents agree to meet the alienating parent and their child at a place where there is video surveillance, such as a petrol station. Although this is intended to prevent any misbehaviour by either parent, sometimes the alienating parent fails to attend or turns up with the child already crying and saying they do not want to see the targeted parent. No one but the alienated parent and their child knows what conversation took place on the journey. The targeted parent is then placed in a situation whereby if they cannot persuade the child to go with them, they have to leave again without them. In this circumstance the targeted parent's position is exploited by the alienating parent, who is in a more powerful position. The impact on the child of this behaviour should be considered, since they will see their alienating parent in control and their targeted parent as vulnerable and/or frustrated and sometimes angry. It is also important to remember that the child is living with the alienating parent and is therefore more likely to align with them.

If children are sent or given gifts by the targeted parent, these are typically rejected and the alienating parent reports that the child did not want them. The alienating parent usually says they attempted to give the gifts to the child. The same behaviours apply to gifts from alienated grandparents or other targeted extended family. Sometimes when court professionals attend the child's home, the gifts can be produced by the alienating parent, who can demonstrate in the presence of the professional person that the child has rejected them. Court professionals are aware that these behaviours can be planned and prepared for, although this can also be the stage when attempts to repair the relationship end, and the alienating parent disrespects the court rulings and fails to support the child to see their targeted parent.

Alienating parents often say the child does not want to attend contact and they do not want to force them to go. When they do this, they are abdicating responsibility for contact onto the child. They are also handing over power when the child may not be mature enough or equipped to manage it. At the same time the child is being encouraged to be cruel towards the targeted parent by rejecting them, and the impact of this behaviour on the child should be a focus of concern. The child is sometimes encouraged to ignore court orders if they are aware of them. It can be stressful for a child who wants to attend contact to have to decline an opportunity to be with their targeted parent in order to please their alienating parent. At already stated, it is usual for the child to live with the alienating parent, and therefore they do not want to do anything that will disrupt their relationship.

Child neglect

In the UK child neglect is said to have occurred when a parent behaves in a manner that is likely to cause unnecessary harm or suffering to a child in their care. In relation to introducing the concept of neglect in cases of PA, it has been noted that parents typically infantilised (treated them as infants or babies) and parentified (the child is required to act as a parent) their child at the same time, and the alienating parent's needs are prioritised (10). This leads to neglect of the child's need to have contact with their other parent and ignores the emotional impact of this on their functioning. There are occasions when this includes leaving the child with other caregivers even when the targeted parent is available.

It has also been found that alienating parents sometimes encourage children not to attend school and neglect their academic needs (12). The alienating parents present as concerned about the child's welfare but have excuses for this behaviour, for example by saying that the school is not meeting the child's needs, or they have medical appointments, or they have health issues which can only be met by the alienating parent at home. In addition, school reports, information and pictures are often not shared with the targeted parent. The targeted parent is in a position whereby they must attempt to nurture their relationships with schoolteachers to ensure they have all the information that they need and can attend parent-teacher meetings separately from the alienating parent.

There are occasions when alienating parents also restrict the child's access to friendship groups and stop them from forming partner relationships. It is believed that this is to prevent any outside influence on the child, although it limits the child's social network and prevents them from becoming independent from the alienating parent (9).

Legal and administrative aggression

Legal and administrative aggression relates to manipulating the legal or other formal systems to cause harm to the targeted parent (13). This often involves making false claims of physical or sexual abuse to the authorities. Unfortunately, this is increasingly common, and targeted parents who are already struggling to cope with conflictual relationships with an ex-partner and a challenging situation with respect to seeing their child might also have to manage allegations of abuse and associated investigations. Children can make untrue allegations of sexual or physical abuse to professionals involved, and this is discussed further in Chapters 4 and 7. Targeted parents have to manage feelings of being misunderstood and judged by others, when in fact they have not carried out the alleged behaviour.

Physical and sexual aggression

Physical and sexual aggression involves either using physical punishment with the child or involving them in sexually inappropriate behaviours if they say they want a relationship with their targeted parent. In the UK it is illegal to leave a mark on a child, and excessive physical intervention can lead to prosecution. Most parents do not admit to using any type of physical punishment, and there have been calls to ban all violent interventions with children (14). In my experience the use of physical discipline is raised occasionally in the context of court reports and has been considered a form of abuse. In these cases, the physical assault has occurred when the alienating parent has not been coping very well with events in their lives, and sadly the child has borne the brunt of their anger.

Other studies that have considered the types of behaviours seen in cases of PA include one carried out in Spain (15). In this study 72 divorced couples were identified through the court system by experts involved in the assessment of intimate partner conflict (domestic violence) (15). It was found 17 alienating behaviours were used by 60% of the alienating parents, and it was reported that in 90% of cases:

- Targeted parents did not receive information about the child.
- Disrespectful behaviours by the child towards the targeted parent were rewarded by the alienating parent.

- The alienating parent made decisions without consulting the targeted parent.
- The alienating parent belittled the targeted parent.
- The alienating parent prevented the targeted parent from visiting the child.

In 80% – 90% of cases, the following strategies were used by the alienating parent:

- Intense questioning after contact (if contact took place).
- Shared information about the court process.
- Interfering in the child's contact with the targeted parent.
- Hindering telephone contact.
- Using other caregivers, without consulting the targeted parent.
- Seeking accomplices, i.e. new partner or extended family.

Other approaches, such as changing the child's address without consulting the targeted parent or trying to change the child's surname, were found in less than 20% of cases of parental alienation.

Having considered what behaviours occur when PA takes place, it is also important to think whether categories of PA could aid an understanding of the concept.

Parental alienation as a form of domestic violence

PA involves a series of behaviours that can have a significant impact on a non-resident parent, their child and their wider family network. More recently, a number of authors have turned their attention to whether parental alienation should be recognised as a form of family violence (10). The argument is that domestic violence (also known as 'intimate partner violence') involves aggressive behaviours or abuse by one partner against another. It can include physical and/or sexual abuse and can present in many different forms, including verbal abuse. Verbal abuse can include emotional manipulation through allegations and negative remarks or by withdrawing from a relationship if the person does not behave as expected. People can have their finances, behaviour, social relationships, emotions and/or other important aspects of life controlled by another individual with whom they are involved. Sometimes people are made to feel as though the abuse is their own fault, and this is sometimes referred to as 'gaslighting'.

Recent authors argue that since the term 'domestic violence' includes an effort to control another's behaviour or emotional welfare through psychological aggression, PA fits under this umbrella term (10). They note that many alienating parents use expressive aggression through derogation, which can be used either overtly or carried out discreetly through playful mocking. In addition, coercive control, which is a means of reducing the power of their partner by controlling their behaviours, is used by limiting access between the parent and child or permitting access only if certain conditions are met.

Parents involved in PA often report each other for every small misdemeanour as they perceive it, for example if a parent is five minutes late for pick-up at contact time or if the child's clothes are dirty when they return from a visit. Sometimes the police are called, and the alienating parent reports violence or simply that they were frightened when the targeted parent arrived to collect their child, even though the contact was arranged through the court, or the alienating parent says the child was abducted by the targeted parent.

Alienating parents who are mothers sometimes claim a male targeted parent is being violent towards them when this is not the case. They can use gender role stereotypes to support their assertions. The alienating parent may say PA is a way to further inflict pain on them when in fact the targeted parent has been totally appropriate in relation to their situation. Sometimes there is a hybrid situation whereby the targeted parent has been angry and has shouted or complained about the behaviour of the alienating parent, which then feeds into their claim that the targeted parent is aggressive. Angry text messages or emails can be shared with legal teams as 'evidence' of the targeted parent's aggressiveness, and in my experience both parents do this.

If a targeted parent is absent due to their employment, this can also be used as a way of hurting them, since the alienating parent can claim that the targeted parent has not spent enough time with the child and does not know them as well as the alienating parent. This is used as a reason for the child not to want to attend contact. If this is true, then it indicates that the alienated child needs to spend more quality time with the targeted parent to help them develop their relationship.

Although it does not occur frequently, there are occasions when the non-resident parent alienates the child (16). Once the child has moved to the care of the alienating parent, they no longer see the targeted parent. In my experience efforts to bring them back together fail, and each time the child begins to show signs of wanting a relationship with the targeted parent, the alienating parent intervenes, and any attempt to reinstate contact breaks down.

Criticisms of the concept of parental alienation

Despite all the evidence gathered from around the world by numerous professionals, some people have written that parental alienation is 'unscientific' and 'an affront to children, women who hold the custody of children of separated couples, science, human rights, and the justice system itself' (17). This is strong language, although interesting because there is an assumption that the resident parent is always female. Of course, today not all resident parents are women, and not all families include a mother and father.

As we will discuss, alienators can be male or female, and although they are mainly female, this is because children mostly reside with their mother after a relationship between a mixed-gender couple ends. Similarly, the parents who are targeted have mostly been male, and this is because fathers have typically left the family home while the children remained in the care of the mother. In my experience, there are *people* who alienate, and their gender is not necessarily the issue;

rather, the emotional harm caused by alienating parents to their children has to be the main focus of the argument.

The term 'parental alienation' has therefore become the foundation of an argument for those who perhaps interpret the term differently to the way it is used today or do not really understand it. Generally, the term 'parental alienation' rather than 'parental alienation syndrome' has become accepted use in practice (18). It seems the prevalence of PA (if we accept the concept) is likely to be higher than recognised, and the associated difficulties are masked and efforts to highlight them are minimised by some. The reality is that until this difficulty is fully recognised and researched, so that an evidence-based understanding of the concept is established, there will continue to be arguments about whether the concept exists. Alienators and their followers or the uninformed argue that it does not happen, but for those who experience it, whether they are parents or children, there is significant damage caused by this issue, which has yet to be elucidated and quantified.

Conclusion

There is already a significant amount of research into the concept of PA, and even when there is an established scientific and research base, it is likely that some people will continue to deny that it happens. We know that there are occasions when parents get into conflictual situations and involve the courts. We know that sometimes one parent makes untrue statements about the other parent or uses other forms of influence to prevent the child from having contact with their (usually non-resident) targeted parent. The issue is becoming commonly known as parental alienation. PA is a form of manipulation which takes place when one parent, usually the resident parent, attempts to influence or succeeds in influencing their children so that they do not wish to have contact with another, usually non-resident, parent. Sometimes the alienating parent's behaviour is supported by grandparents, extended family and/or friends. PA is a process and does not usually happen as a single event. In most cases, it involves two parents who have separated, leaving the children in the care of one parent. Often the parent who is leaving the home had a good relationship with the child or children before the relationship with the other parent ended. Sometimes the targeted parent left the family when the mother was pregnant or just after the baby was born, before the child and targeted parent had an opportunity to develop a relationship. In cases where a relationship had formed, the parent who has left the family, gradually or sometimes suddenly, finds the relationship with the children diminishes or ends. In most instances, the alienating parent states that the child does not want to go to contact, and the targeted parent is confused about what has happened. Cases where there really are justifiable reasons for the child not wanting to go to contact are not PA. Sometimes the targeted parent believes that the child is 'going through a phase', waits for the child to adjust to the relationship ending and hopes that their behaviour will change if they just retreat for a while. In my experience, a targeted parent's decision to 'back off' for a period of time usually happens on the advice of another person, sometimes a professional. There are also occasions when the alienating parent tells them this is what they need to do. Although it cannot be ruled out that the alienating parent believes this, there are also occasions when the alienating parent is intent on causing a disturbance in the targeted parent/ child relationship without thinking, knowing or sometimes even caring about the impact on the children of removing a parent from their lives.

References

1 Harman, J.J., Bernet, W. and Harman, J. (2019). Parental alienation: The blossoming of a field of study. *Current Directions in Psychological Science*, 1–6.
2 Tavares, A., Crespo, C. and Ribeiro, M.T. (2021). What does it mean to be a targeted parent? Parents' experiences in the context of parental alienation. *Journal of Child and Family Studies*. doi:10.1007/s10826-21-01914-6.
3 Baker, A.J.L. and Chambers, J. (2011). Adult recall of childhood exposure to parental conflict: Unpacking the black box of parental alienation. *Journal of Divorce and Remarriage*, 52, 55–76.
4 Warshak, R.A. (2019). When evaluators get it wrong: False positives IDs and parental alienation. *Psychology, Public Policy and Law*, 26, 54–68. doi:10.1037/law0000216.
5 Office for National Statistics. (2019). www.Ons.gov.uk Families and Households in the UK 2019.
6 Harman, J.J., Leder-Elder, S. and Biringer, Z. (2019). Prevalence of adults who are the targets of parental alienating behaviors and their impact. *Children and Youth Services Review*, 106. doi:10.1016/j.childyouth.2019.104471.
7 Hands, A.J. and Warshak, R.A. (2011). Parental alienation among college students. *The American Journal of Family Therapy*, 39, 431–443. http://dx.doi.org/10/1080/109 26187.2011.575336.
8 Ben-Ami, N. and Baker, A.J.L. (2012). The long-term correlates of childhood exposure to parental alienation on adult self-sufficiency and well-being. *The American Journal of Family Therapy*, 40, 169–283.
9 Baker, A.J.L. and Darnall, D. (2006). Behaviours and strategies of parental alienation: A survey of parental experiences. *Journal of Divorce and Remarriage*, 45, 55–76. doi:10.1300/J087v45n01_06.
10 Harman, J.J., Kruk, E. and Hines, D.A. (2018). Parental alienating behaviors: An unacknowledged form of family violence. *Psychological Bulletin*, 144, 1275–1299. doi:10.1037/bu10000175.
11 Garber, B.D. (2011). Parental alienation and the dynamics of the enmeshed parent-child dyad: Adultification, parentification and infantilization. *Family Court Review*, 49, 322–335.
12 Harman, J.J. and Biringen, Z. (2016). *Parents acting badly: How institutions and societies promote the alienation of children from their loving families*. Fort Collins: Colorado Parental Alienation Project, LLC.
13 Hines, D.A., Douglas, E.M. and Berger, J.L. (2015). A self-report measure of legal and administrative aggression within intimate relationships. *Aggressive Behavior*, 41, 295–309. doi:10.1002/ab.21540.

14 Freeman, M. and Saunders, B.J. (2014). Can we conquer child abuse if we don't outlaw physical chastisement of children? *The International Journal of Children's Rights*, 22, 681–709. doi:10.1163/15718182-012204002.

15 López, T.J., Iglesias, V.E.N. and García, P.F. (2014). Parental alienation gradient: Strategies for a syndrome. *The American Journal of Family Therapy*, 42, 217–231. doi:10.1080/01926187.2013.820116.

16 Warshak, R.A. (2015). Ten parental alienation fallacies that compromise decisions in court and in therapy. *Professional Psychology, Research and Practice*, 46, 235–249.

17 Clemente, M. and Padilla-Racero, D. (2016). When courts accept what science rejects: Custody issues concerning the alleged 'parental alienation syndrome'. *Journal of Child Custody*, 13, 126–133. doi:10.1080/15379418.2016.1219245.

18 Boch-Galhau, W. (2018). Parental alienation (syndrome) – A serious form of psychological child abuse. *Mental Health and Family Medicine*, 14, 725–739.

Chapter 3

Mild, moderate and severe parental alienation

Introduction

Parental alienation occurs after separation and involves one parent interrupting or attempting to interfere with a child's relationship with their other parent, inducing a negative response in the child towards the targeted parent. Five behaviours have been found to be present in 90% of cases: (a) failure to share information with the targeted parent about the child; (b) rewarding disrespectful behaviour by the child towards the targeted parent; (c) denigrating the targeted parent in front of the child; (d) failing to involve the targeted parent when making important decisions about the child and (e) obstructing attendance at contact (1). The extent and impact of the interference depends on many factors, and attempts have been made to try to categorise PA into mild, moderate and severe alienation (2–3). This is an effort to try to help understand the difficulties and promote appropriate signposting to intervention if needed.

Mild parental alienation

Mild PA can be very subtle and may begin during the parents' separation process. This means it can begin to occur slowly over a number of years. For example, the alienating parent may frown and/or hesitate when they speak about the targeted parent, indicating that they do not have a positive opinion of them, or they may have pressure of speech, sound anxious and suggest that the targeted parent presents as a threat. The child may notice the behaviours of the alienating parent more than the content of speech (4). The alienating parent may grumble about the targeted parent's behaviour or their parenting ability but not usually in a sustained manner. Several authors have found that some strategies for alienation are used more frequently than others, and belittling the targeted parent in the presence of the child was a behaviour carried out by many alienating parents (1, 5).

In mild PA the alienating parent might denigrate the targeted parent at times, although this does not tend to be sustained. At this stage both parents enable the child to hold their own opinion of events. The child is supported by the alienating parent to attend contact. The child typically turns up and engages with the targeted

DOI: 10.4324/9781003156147-3

parent in their usual manner when the alienating parent is absent. Sometimes this happens shortly after parental separation, when the alienating parent is still recovering. Once the family has recovered from the separation, the relationship between the child and targeted parent is permitted to return to normal, and alienation stops. Sadly, at other times, depending on the personalities and circumstances involved, mild alienation proceeds to become moderate.

In cases of mild PA, although the child may criticise the targeted parent, once they are with them, it is as if the criticism never happened (4). Although they may be hesitant at the beginning of any contact session, over time they engage more fully. Generally, when they are not with the alienating parent, the child enjoys their time with the targeted parent and engages with them as if the denigration or other alienating behaviours never happened. If the PA progresses, then sometimes during this stage the child may begin to change the way they feel toward the targeted parent, and this may be reinforced by the alienating parent rewarding any negativity towards the targeted parent. Some children begin to feel unhappy at this time, and this may be manifested by behavioural disturbance and attributed to the impact of divorce. The child loves both their parents but is unable to express this openly and gradually begins to withdraw emotionally from the targeted parent. Any change in the child's behaviour tends to be almost indiscernible to the targeted parent, who can feel that something may have changed in the way the child behaves towards them but cannot quite identify it.

Meanwhile the alienating parent may refuse the child when they ask to make calls to the targeted parent or request to spend more time with them. The child may be refused requests to purchase birthday or other celebratory cards for the targeted parent or their extended family. The child may feel pulled towards the alienating parent without having awareness that this is occurring. The child may sense tension when the alienating parent refers to the targeted parent and may begin to feel that they are disloyal to the alienating parent or making them unhappy when they spend time with their other parent. Given that the alienating parent is now usually their main carer, this can begin to feel a little uncomfortable for the child. At this stage, the child may either agree with any negative comments made about the targeted parent by the alienating parent, or the child may criticise the targeted parent themselves. The allegations can present as irrational or unreasonable. The child may begin to say they do not always wish to attend contact, and although initially the targeted parent may not wish to over-interpret events, they begin to see the gradual emotional withdrawal of their child and wonder whether their ex-partner is influential in this behaviour.

Thoughts about their child not wanting to spend time with them can be very anxiety-provoking for the targeted parent, particularly as they do not usually see the child every day to assess the situation themselves. If asked whether their child could miss contact for one week, they might dismiss their own thoughts or concerns and try to remain child-focused; after all, 'what's one contact session if the child wishes to attend a birthday party'? Sometimes it is true that a child wishes to attend an event when contact is due to take place, and it is therefore important for the absent parent to manage any anxiety and avoid jumping to conclusions when a request of this nature is made. It is also important that they do not offload any emotional response about this situation to either the child or the alienating parent as it will make them appear unreasonable and difficult. At the same time, it is important that an alienating parent does not present as pleased in the presence of a targeted parent if the child declines contact, and if they do, the targeted parent needs to try to manage this without verbal retaliation. The targeted parent needs to withhold any negative thoughts about the child or the alienating parent's behaviour in these circumstances. Repeated cancellations can be a sign of alienation.

As already said, it is usually the case that targeted and alienating parents have not separated on good terms, and therefore any lack of trust between them facilitates bad feeling on both sides. The targeted parent can begin to feel anxious about any lack of contact or change in the child when they see them (even though a child can change quite rapidly due to influences outside of the family). When contact has been cancelled several times, this can begin to impact on the relationship between the child and their targeted parent. As a child develops, their interests change, and the targeted parent can quickly fall out of step with their child's needs. As the targeted parent does not live with their child, they do not see them every day to know about their school events or friendship dramas. It is easy for a parent to become out of sync with their child's needs.

When a parent is trying to engage with a child they do not know well or have an easy relationship with, it can be stressful for all involved. A stressed parent can mistakenly be overly zealous with discipline or irritable and argumentative. This does nothing to improve the relationship with their child. Episodes of angst can be stressful for the child, who in turn hesitates to commit to further contact. This can create a vicious cycle of uncertainty, and a lack of enthusiasm from either side can easily be misinterpreted when there is an emotional attachment between the parties, particularly as each side is concerned about being hurt. The child is then reluctant to participate in reconciliation, preferring to remain at home, where they know the rules and do not have the stress of getting things wrong. This situation can easily be exploited by the alienating parent.

There are findings that sometimes a child will attempt to discuss feelings of disengagement with an alienating parent's extended family (4). As grandparents are often involved in alienation, they may reinforce any negative opinions held about the targeted parent or their extended family.

It is also the case that after parents separate their circumstances often change, and this can lead to a situation whereby the rules for contact need to be modified. If the parents change their communication style after their separation resulting from their experiences, then this can lead to misunderstandings, and alienation can result. The alienating parent may not be aware initially of the impact of their behaviour on their child. A mildly alienating parent might be upset if the targeted parent meets a new partner or if they are overwhelmed by the experience of lone parenting. They might convey this inappropriately through lack of emotional regulation, although they are likely to later reflect, feel guilty and express remorse for their behaviours and explain to their child their circumstances and feelings. Similarly, targeted parents may express negative emotion and later regret comments or accusations made, but the situation can usually be resolved if an apology is made and the child is made aware of the targeted parent's emotional welfare. To prevent further alienation, both parents need to make their child aware that they are able to love their parents without exposure to further interference. Parents need to focus on ensuring their child has an optimum experience, rather than dragging them into any residual emotional quagmire. This offers parents an opportunity to create an exciting new situation with their child that can be enjoyed by everyone involved. This will improve the child's bonds with their parents and ensure they have the best chance for achieving their potential in their academic, social and home lives.

Mild alienation does not help the child to manage any emotions associated with one parent moving out of the family home and any other change in their circumstances. When parents separate, children typically do not have any say in the matter and often do not choose who they will live with or how often they will see their absent parent. Depending on the age of the child, it is important to recognise that the child has thoughts and feelings about their situation, too, and they cannot be expected to accept what the parents have decided is the best situation for them without being able to make a contribution and express their opinion. If the parents do not agree with the child's suggestions about contact, they can then explain to them, in a positive way that does not cause them emotional distress, why decisions have been made. In doing this, children learn that their opinion matters and that they are respected, and if changes need to be made, the child can be consulted. They also learn how to negotiate in relationships and how to manage themselves by the parents' example. Parents can become role models and demonstrate to their children how to resolve disputes and promote positive exchanges in complex situations.

Mild PA can develop into moderate PA and also into severe PA and it could be argued they are on a continuum. Categories are helpful as they create boundaries for intervention proposals. The mildly alienating parent typically responds well to education, as they want to meet their child's needs and are concerned about offering optimum parenting support and opportunity. Early intervention by way of psychoeducation is key to prevent the situation from deteriorating further, which then requires professional help.

Moderate Parental Alienation

Although it is not always the case, moderate alienation often begins to creep in after a parent meets a new partner. The new partner might be referred to as 'dad' or 'mum' and may attend parenting appointments with the resident parent, essentially filling the role that the other parent previously held. At this stage a parent can begin to feel more powerful as they have support for any alienating behaviour. Sometimes a new partner encourages or even instigates alienation behaviours as they do not want the previous partner in their lives. The alienating parent may not make the targeted parent aware of school events or issues relating to their child. The child then is in a situation with a 'new' parent who presents as very invested in their welfare and a targeted parent who appears not to care. There might be suggestions to move to a new house or area, and if the child is excited about these suggestions and they are not supported by the targeted parent, then the child might perceive this negatively. The child sometimes idolises the alienating parent's new partner, whilst at the same time saying that the targeted parent does not make them happy.

Moderate parental alienation is typically seen during handovers (6). The alienating parent's denigration of the targeted parent is obvious at this time, and some of the signs of the more severe cases begin to creep in. For example, the child is less ambivalent than they were previously, and they are beginning to describe the alienating parent as 'all good' and the targeted parent as 'all bad'. The child is reluctant to attend contact and usually must be persuaded to go, although they gradually engage with the targeted parent once they are no longer with the alienating parent.

At this stage, the child begins to protect the alienating parent and asserts that their claims about the targeted parent are their own. They appear to be oblivious to any hurt they may cause the targeted parent, begin to make comments about the targeted parent's extended family and present as reluctant to see them. They begin to see the alienating parent, their extended family and partner as 'all good' and the targeted family, their extended family and partner as 'all bad'. They start using 'borrowed scenarios', which are situations described by other adults in their lives that portray the targeted parent negatively and usually involve violence or poor behaviour. The child has typically listened to these events and processed them in a way that shows their targeted parent in a poor light. Some children do not have the cognitive ability or maturity to recognise what is happening, and they begin to align themselves with the alienating parent, which presents a significantly less stressful option than trying to continue their relationship with the targeted parent in the face of opposition from several adults.

Sometimes the alienating parent tells the child that the targeted parent's behaviour reflects a lack of care or love, which can impact on a child's self-esteem and/ or make them feel angry. The child might begin to feel that the targeted parent abandoned them, and they are fortunate to have the alienating parent to take care of them. If the targeted parent becomes irritated by the alienating parent's behaviour, they can contribute to the problem by getting into conflict with them or by being tense or rigid with the child. If the targeted parent criticises the alienating parent to the child, this contributes to the child's feelings of confusion. Some targeted parents withdraw from contact. Often this is because they are concerned about the impact of conflict on the child. This can support any allegations made by the alienating parent that relate to the targeted parent's lack of commitment to the child.

It is possible that the child may have a personality type that leads to their feeling more comfortable and secure with the targeted parent. The targeted parent might offer more stability and a wider family network that the child has previously engaged happily with. This can lead the child to feel very conflicted when they are asked to deny these feelings and align themselves with the alienated parent. These feelings can be very difficult for the child to cope with, leading to behavioural disturbance and greater reluctance to go to contact, since handovers and collections are so emotionally loaded and tense (6–7).

At this stage the alienating parent might begin to introduce some thoughts about what the child might be missing when they attend contact, so they suggest that whilst the child was absent, they had an interesting time and engaged with activities that the child was likely to have enjoyed. They talk about these events a lot and suggest to the child that they missed out by not being part of it. If there are younger half or stepsiblings, they are also included in the process. Interesting events with the targeted parent are minimised, and the alienating parent fails to reinforce any joy the child experiences that results from these. The alienating parent usually avoids speaking about the targeted parent, and if they do say something it is rarely positive. Pictures or reminders of the targeted parent are not evident in the home. Indirect attacks are made on the targeted parent and their extended family by comments that can be interpreted as innocuous if they are repeated. For example, sometimes the alienating parent asks the child whether they would like to spend time on holiday when the child is scheduled to see the targeted parent, making it difficult for them to say no. Or they book a trip that clashes with a period when the child is supposed to be with the targeted parent, making the child appear difficult if they raise this as an issue.

The alienating parent can also at this stage begin to introduce inappropriate information to the child, for example, that their targeted parent hurt them emotionally by becoming involved with someone else or by leaving them, breaking a promise when they said they would always be together. The alienating parent also introduces information about the court process, noting that it is a negative and unnecessary experience for them and associating the court process with the targeted parent's behaviour, rather than their own. The child does not understand that the reason the targeted parent has gone to court is usually because the alienating parent is blocking their relationship, and that in doing so, they are demonstrating commitment to the child, rather than attempting to harm the alienating parent.

As children get older, they notice differences in financial status. If the targeted parent appears affluent and the alienating parent is not, then this can be used against them and the alienating parent is the victim. Similarly, if the reverse is true, this can be because the targeted parent did not work hard enough. Whatever the situation, it can be perceived in such a way as to make the alienating parent the victim and the targeted parent the aggressor, despite the opposite holding true.

The parent might begin to interfere with contact, either by telling the child what they are to expect during contact or by giving the child things to do when they are with their targeted parent. The alienating parent might tell the child to ring or text them if there are any problems, laying the groundwork for the child to feel that problems might arise. They may also send food or money, indicating that the targeted parent will not meet the child's needs. The alienating parent might also ring or text the child to check their welfare during contact. This suggests to the child that their alienating parent is concerned about their welfare whilst they are with the targeted parent. The alienating parent is unlikely to want to hear that the situation is good, and so the child is required to minimise their experiences for the alienating parent's benefit.

It is reported that at this stage the child begins to feel responsible for the welfare of their alienating parent (8). They do not express empathy for the targeted parent and do not understand that their situation is likely to contribute to any poor behaviours observed. The impact of this on the child's personality has to be considered, since they are learning that it is okay to be unkind to others.

When there is justifiable estrangement in addition to alienation and a hybrid situation occurs, this offers an opportunity to the alienating parent which can be exploited to support their case. Any poor behaviour on the part of the targeted parent can be recorded and shared with legal teams and other professionals and will throw doubt on assertions from the targeted parent that they are reasonable and a victim of alienating behaviour. Although it might be difficult for both parents to understand their contribution to their situation, it is important for them to receive education about the impact of their behaviours on the child. This is covered in Chapters 10 and 11 on interventions.

When there are siblings, if one is influenced by the alienating parent, they can apply pressure to their (usually younger) brothers or sisters to ensure they are not free to fully enjoy the contact session either. This means siblings are concerned about enjoying contact in the event that this might be reported back to the alienating parent.

Despite all this, and although the child expresses a lack of desire to see the targeted parent, with moderate alienation they continue to demonstrate some flexibility in thinking and can be talked around. Although there may be signs of reluctance to attend, there continues to be some contact, and the child presents as enjoying themselves with the targeted parent. The child's mood might fluctuate during the visit, so that they are initially reluctant before engaging in a more relaxed manner, then become more anxious and irritable towards the end of the contact period when they know they have to encounter the alienating parent's behaviours again. It is important for the targeted parent not to denigrate any aspect of the child's life with the alienating parent or their new circumstances and also to allow the child to be tense and/or irritable when they are leaving. It is possible the child may feel sad about leaving the targeted parent and/or anxious about returning to the care of an alienating parent who may quiz them about their time away. Framing this as a sign of loss can be sad for a targeted parent, but it is unhelpful to the child if they too become stressed about the upcoming separation at the end of contact. It is important for the targeted parent to model appropriate behaviour by focusing on the positive aspects of the next contact session and also by making the transition back to the alienating parent as comfortable as possible for their child.

In relation to the specific task of reuniting the child with their targeted parent after a period of separation, there are many parenting programmes available for those who wish to work collaboratively to provide the best possible experience for their child under the circumstances. People can also be court-mandated to attend these courses, and there is a hope, then, that they will learn from them and move forward in a more positive manner. Sometimes even moderate cases of PA can gain benefit from parenting courses or family therapy, and the family can learn to recognise the problems for the child in managing different sets of rules in different homes, and the parents can try to accept that their child may need some time to adjust when they return from the other parent's home, and this does not necessarily reflect a poor contact experience. The child may present as different to the way they were when the parent last saw them, but the child will need time to adjust between homes. Also, the child is developing, and as they get older, they will also be influenced by their peer group. Sometimes a combination of influence from another home and their peer group can lead the child to behave in new ways that a parent can find alien, and everyone has to adjust to a new set of behaviours or attitudes. Often, a child will modify their behaviour for each home as time goes on, much in the way they would if they visited grandparents' or friends' homes where different rules apply.

Severe parental alienation

The severely alienated child does not usually see their targeted parent, and although they are likely to have had a good relationship in the past, over time this has changed. The severely alienated child may not have seen their targeted parent for many years. Their history together has been re-written by the alienated child and contrasts sharply with videos or pictures produced by the targeted parent that often show a giggling or laughing child in the care of the targeted parent during happier times. Videos sometimes show the child sitting on the targeted parent's lap or playing with their hair or generally being affectionate, yet the targeted child will claim that they do not remember these events or that the targeted parent has doctored the information to make it appear more positive than the child felt at the time. The child will often say that they were unhappy when the video or pictures were taken, no matter how it looks. The child is very difficult to negotiate with and usually has a mantra about the targeted parent and their extended family. Children who identify as female and adolescents have been found to be more likely to be severely alienated. It was noted that in the latter set of circumstances, this is likely to be because alienating parents have had more time to expose their child to alienating behaviours (5).

The severely alienated child often makes significant allegations against the targeted parent, which sometimes includes sexual assault. These allegations can result in many police and professional interviews for the child, as well as intrusive examinations. The child is adamant that these events took place, and no evidence is found. Experienced professionals typically find the interviews to be bizarre and not in keeping with the information shared by other children who are making similar allegations. These allegations do a disservice to children who have actually been sexually assaulted, as they undermine the seriousness of this crime and the emotional consequences which can be lifelong. Other allegations often relate to violence against the alienated child and/or their parent. Usually when asked for detail, the information given is inconsistent, even over the course of the interview, and sometimes it makes no sense at all. Sometimes the child describes events they could not possibly remember that happened shortly after they were born.

The severely alienated child treats their targeted parent with extreme hostility (9). When they are spoken to about their targeted parent, they often present as angry and can express strong dislike of them. At times they threaten to harm the severely targeted parent and say they wish to remove them from the alienating parent's life. Threats can be extreme and include killing the targeted parent and their extended family. The level of emotion and distress exhibited by the severely alienated child when their targeted parent is mentioned can be very upsetting for professionals and can include shouting and crying and hiding. The presentation can lead to unnecessary referrals to mental health services, and the child can then present as calm and collected, so professionals are confused about why they have been referred.

Often the court decides that severely alienated children should receive gifts and cards by way of indirect contact. These are shared via the targeted and alienating parents' solicitors so that they can be examined for appropriateness and also to support the targeted parent's assertions that the items were sent (as sometimes alienating parents will say that gifts have not been received). When they arrive with the alienated child, several outcomes are possible. When the solicitor is not present, the alienating parent can put the gifts and cards into the bin without the alienated child ever knowing they were given. More often the alienating parent retains the items in the event that a legal professional, such as the court children's officer or a social worker, might ask to see them later. When they are asked about them, the alienating parent claims that they attempted to give them to the alienated child, but the child refused to accept them. The alienating parent can produce the gifts/cards and ask the court professional to see the child's reaction for themselves. It appears that the child is usually aware that this is likely to occur, and they sometimes refuse to even look at the items. Alternatively, the child claims the targeted parent bought them items they did not want, even though the court has checked with the alienating parent beforehand to ensure the correct gifts were purchased. The alienating child can tear up a card from the targeted parent or refuse to listen if it is read to them by a legal professional. Sometimes they listen and then say confidently that they do not want the gift, or it is the wrong gift, or that they simply do not wish to see their targeted parent and they do not know why the parent keeps trying to contact them. Sometimes severely alienated children make statements that are very similar or the same as the ones the alienating parent made about the targeted parent. This includes the use of adult language that would not usually be in the vocabulary of a child of their age. Rather than support the alienating parent's assertions that the targeted parent is the problem, this completely undermines them and provides evidence of alienating behaviours.

Severely alienated children can present 'normally' with their alienated parent and others, such as teachers; however, some are so damaged they are angry with everyone and are brought to mental health or other services (9). The alienating parent usually says any poor behaviour results from the targeted parent's continued insistence that they should have contact. It is reported that children are less frequently filled with fear than hatred, but there are occasions when they genuinely appear to believe that their targeted parent presents as a threat to them. This causes them significant anxiety, and at times they are unable to function effectively. This has led to concerns about how cruel it is to instill unnecessary fear into a child (9).

Severe alienation is cruel to both the child and the targeted parent, and although the alienating parent appears oblivious to this, it hurts everyone involved, including themselves at times. It has been argued that rejecting a parent unreasonably is as significant a problem as other irrational aversions and anxieties, and severe alienation impacts on a child's cognitive, emotional and behavioural development (9). For the targeted parent, they can feel as though their child is lost to them forever, and there are occasions when this happens. In addition, every year a parent and child are apart, they are both missing out on the opportunity for the targeted parent to attend school concerts, formals, sports matches, music recitals and other significant life events, such as graduations. The child will be aware of their targeted parent's absence, even if they have a new 'mum' or 'dad' present.

In severe cases of PA some alienating parents as well as some targeted parents and some children involved have mental health problems. However, whilst PA can be a sign of emotional disturbance or difficulty adjusting to a new set of circumstances, sometimes pathologising issues is less helpful than accepting that each case has individual needs. That is why education for all professionals is so important for those likely to come into contact with PA.

Conclusion

Attempts have been made to categorise PA as 'mild', 'moderate' or 'severe'. These are a helpful way for professionals to understand what to expect in a particular situation and also explain the process that the alienated child is likely to be exposed to. Mild alienation might be carried out obliviously by the alienating parent and can usually be changed relatively easily without significant intervention. Moderate alienation usually indicates that the alienating parent knows what they are doing and has decided to continue. Typically, severe alienation follows moderate alienating behaviours, and it is rare for the child to see the targeted parent at this stage. Sometimes with severe alienation allegations of physical and/or sexual abuse of the child and/or the alienating parent are made. It is usually the case that if there is more than one child in a family, they will be alienated gradually and will not all stop attending contact at the same time.

References

1   López, T.J., Iglesias, V.E.N. and García, P.F. (2014). Parental alienation gradient: Strategies for a syndrome. *The American Journal of Family Therapy*, 42, 217–231. doi:10.1080/01926187.2013.820116.
2   Gardner, R.A., Sauber, S.R. and Lorandos, D. (Eds.). (2006). *The international handbook of parental alienation syndrome: Conceptual, clinical and legal considerations*. Springfield, IL: Charles C. Thomas Publisher.
3   Lorandos, D., Bernet, W. and Sauber, S.R. (Eds.). (2013). *Parental alienation: The handbook for mental health and legal professionals*. Springfield, IL: Charles C. Thomas Publisher.
4   Darnell, D.C. (2013). Mild cases of parental alienation. In D. Lorendos, W. Bernet and S.R. Sauber (Eds.), *American series in behavioural science and law: Parental alienation: The handbook for mental health and legal professionals* (pp. 74–96). Springfield, IL: Charles C. Thomas Publisher.
5   Baker, A.J.L. and Darnell, D. (2006). Behaviours and strategies employed in parental alienation: A survey of parental experiences. *Journal of Divorce and Remarriage*, 45, 97–124. doi:10.1300/J087v45n01_06.
6   Worenklein, A. (2013). Moderate cases of parental alienation. In D. Lorendos, W. Bernet and S.R. Sauber (Eds.), *American series in behavioural science and law: Parental alienation: The handbook for mental health and legal professionals* (pp. 74–96). Springfield, IL: Charles C. Thomas Publisher.
7   Warshak, R.A. (2020). Risks and realities of working with alienated children. *Family Court Review*, 58(2), 432–455.
8   Baker, A.J.L. (2007). *Adult children of parental alienation syndrome: Breaking the ties that bind*. New York: W.W. Norton.
9   Warshak, R.A. (2013). Severe cases of parental alienation. In D. Lorendos, W. Bernet and S.R. Sauber (Eds.), *American series in behavioural science and law: Parental alienation: The handbook for mental health and legal professionals* (pp. 74–96). Springfield, IL: Charles C. Thomas Publisher.

Chapter 4

Fallacies, hybrid cases and justifiable estrangement

Introduction

Parental alienation occurs when one parent manipulates a child against their other parent, and use of the term assumes the other parent has not behaved in a way that justifies the alienating parent's behaviour (this is discussed further later), although court experts can become confused, particularly when they encounter their first PA case. This is because PA behaviours run counter to the way experts are typically trained to expect during assessment. These cases are often characterised by high levels of social desirability, general unreliability of the information presented and difficulty for experts in establishing the facts. Many cases involve a 'hybrid' situation whereby one parent is alienating the child and the second parent has also behaved inappropriately and has contributed to the problem. There are also occasions when the estrangement between a child and a parent are justified, for example if a parent is unable to control their aggression and presents as a risk to the child. The various situations that occur can lead to a misinterpretation by a court expert, and associated with this, inappropriate advice can be offered.

Fallacies

Ten fallacies about PA have been identified that influence decision-making in court (1–2). It has been noted that frequent repetition of incorrect information can lead to a situation whereby it is believed to be true, even if this is not the case (1). The ten fallacies are:

1   **A child will not unreasonably reject a parent with whom they spend most of their time**. It has been noted that although a child can be helped to reinstate a relationship with an absent parent by spending more time with them, it is not the case that a child cannot be alienated from a parent when they spend more time with them than they do with an alienating parent. This situation often arises when a parent alienates a child from their other parent during contact. The resident parent can become targeted without their having any idea that this is taking place. Warshak reports he has seen more than 50 cases in which a father (he specifically said fathers) alienated a child during

DOI: 10.4324/9781003156147-4

contact, and the child had complied mostly either because they were afraid of upsetting the father or because they felt the father needed them (1). This situation has also presented itself during my clinical practice, although it is significantly less common than alienation by the resident parent.

2 **A child will not unreasonably reject their mother.** This belief fails to recognise the extent of influence one adult can have over their child. A number of studies have found PA alienators to be between one-third and one-half-male (1, 3–6). Most of the studies do not consider situations in which there are two mothers or both parents are fathers, and these have yet to be considered.

3 **Parents contribute equally to alienation.** There are situations where both parents contribute equally to parental alienation, but these are not associated with 'pure' PA behaviours; rather these typically result from a 'hybrid' situation (1). In PA the alienating parent is responsible for the emotional abuse of the child due to their behaviour, and the targeted parent's contribution is minimal or non-existent. For example, formerly alienated children who have reunited with their targeted parent have changed their view of the targeted parent in the context of more information and insight into their alienation (1).

4 **Alienation is a temporary response to parental separation.** This can lead to a situation whereby a well-meaning therapist supports a child to 'wait until they have recovered' before attempting to re-engage with their other parent. Typically, this means the child does not have contact with their targeted parent and therefore does not reunite with them.

5 **Parental rejection can be a healthy coping strategy after separation.** The assumption is that the child wishes to exercise control over their situation and chooses not to see the targeted parent, and by doing so they avoid torn loyalties. It is therefore important that courts intervene and order contact, so that children do not have the burden of assuming responsibility for choices they make, particularly if they have to challenge one parent's wishes.

6 **A young child living with an alienating parent does not require intervention.** It is recognised that a small child who acts in a fearful manner in the presence of a targeted parent is likely to become more entrenched if no intervention takes place (1). If the child receives intervention by way of opportunity to enjoy time with the targeted parent, then any frightened and aversive behaviour dissipates (7–8). Alienated children often need assistance by way of knowing they are permitted to enjoy contact with their targeted parent.

7 **Alienated adolescents should be permitted to make decisions about their contact.** It is sometimes felt that teenagers have the cognitive capacity to make their own decisions about contact, and also it can be very difficult to try to enforce any decision-making in favour of their having contact with a targeted parent. This ignores the fact that the child might have been influenced many years before they made their decision and grown up holding a negative view of the targeted parent. It also assumes that teenagers cannot be influenced by an alienating parent. This also ignores the fact that teenagers remain under the control of others with respect to their education, alcohol use, ability to drive, get married, etc.

8 **An alienating child who is functioning well in other areas of life does not require intervention.** Some believe that if a child is doing well in other areas of life, such as in their academic world, then no intervention is required. This approach does not recognise that the presentation can be superficial and that difficulties can be hidden; for example, problems with peers or alcohol/drug use can be undisclosed. Growing up thinking it is reasonable to mistreat the other parent can impact on peer relations, or avoidance of troubling thoughts can lead to alcohol/drug use. Also, if the alienated child is enmeshed with the alienating parent, they can feel responsible for the alienating parent's emotional state, comfort them and reassure them of their allegiance, and not indicate their true thoughts or feelings.

9 **Therapeutic intervention will be successful even if the child lives with their alienating parent.** Therapeutic intervention to try to improve the child's relationship with their targeted parent cannot be helpful if there is an effort to undermine it by the alienating parent. It is likely to lead to further confusion for any child involved. There are no outcome studies to show effectiveness, and some research indicates that intervention makes the situation worse (9–10). Overall, outcome studies show no change if the child continues not to see their targeted parent.

10 **Separating the child from the alienating parent is traumatic.** No peer-reviewed publication has demonstrated children are harmed by removal from an alienating parent. Within the studies considered for this book, no adult who was removed to the care of a targeted parent during childhood has later declared regret about the move. Studies of adults who were alienated as children found they expressed guilt and sadness about having to reject a parent (11). Suggestions of trauma and evocative language from an alienating parent are based on their own emotional response to the situation rather than thinking about what is best for their child. If the alienating parent was able to prioritise the child, the child would have had contact with their targeted parent before professionals began to talk about removal.

There are situations when PA is referred to but may not actually be occurring (2). Many of those who object to the term 'parental alienation' focus on those situations; however, court experts who are genuinely interested in supporting families in which PA occurs recognise the differences between a genuine case of PA and one where there are a number of factors likely to explain the family's presentation. These factors are then considered when recommendations are being made to the court. These include:

•   When a court expert over-values one aspect of an alienating parent's behaviour, such as shouting as 'evidence' of alienation.
•   A child's temporary behaviour is misinterpreted as alienation when the child usually has a positive relationship with their non-resident parent but has withdrawn for a particular reason, e.g. following a disagreement.

Hybrid situations

Hybrid situations occur when there are both rational and irrational reasons for a child not having contact with their nonpreferred parent. If there is a mix between alienating behaviours by one parent and the targeted parent behaving in a way that has contributed to the child's decision not to engage with them, this is known as a hybrid case. This situation can occur when a child has mixed feelings about their nonpreferred parent and so presents with some coherent and rational reasons for rejecting them, as well as some irrational and troubled ideas that do not make sense (12). As a hybrid situation can be difficult to understand and disentangle, it is important for assessors to attempt to elucidate the reasons why a child says they do not want to see their parent in the context of a favoured parent's behaviour. Examples might include the situation whereby a child is predisposed to prefer one parent and has clashed with the other parent in the past, or the targeted parent has some difficulty with drug/alcohol use or mental health issues, or they have caused the child to feel disappointed in the past. The latter does not refer to occasions when a parent has been unpredictably detained and apologised for being late, or accidentally disappointed the child, but rather when they have been careless. It is reasonable for the child to feel upset in these cases and perhaps express concern about attending contact.

There are occasions when a combination of events results in a child not having contact with their non-preferred parent. The child may hold a contradictory view of the non-preferred parent; some of these are justified and reasonable, and others are not and do not explain the child's animosity. This can result in the belief that a preferred parent is responsible for the child's relationship with their nonpreferred parent, when in fact other factors are contributing.

Children can be critical of their parents at times, but this does not typically result in rejection. If a child focuses on the negative aspects of their nonpreferred parent's behaviour or personality and the preferred parent does not support them to understand what is going on, then the child may reject the nonpreferred parent, and the result is a hybrid situation whereby both parents have contributed. For example, this might occur if the nonpreferred parent expected the child to enjoy contact on their terms but did not listen to the child's desires or wishes or if the nonpreferred parent denigrated the preferred parent during contact. These issues can result in the child not wishing to spend time with their nonpreferred parent. It has been reported that although children sometimes refuse to see their targeted parent shortly after the parental separation, this does not mean they will never see them again, only that they are adjusting to their new situation (2). Other situations might suggest PA when it is not occurring:

- A child may experience emotional disturbance, which may or may not be associated with the parental separation. If they did not want their parents to separate, they might decide to punish them by rejection, and in these circumstances, they might also punish the resident parent.

- A child might be reluctant to leave a parent who needs emotional support and may need reassurance from them in order to be able to leave.
- The child resists contact because they do not like the parent's new environment, group of friends, family situation, etc. This is particularly the case if the parent ignores or minimises the contact as a result of needing to meet the demands of other parties.
- The child feels closer to one parent, and the other parent feels threatened by this and is demanding as a result.
- The child is more comfortable in one parent's home. This is most likely to occur if the child is unhappy with the parenting style of one parent, or they might prefer to be with the more emotionally sensitive parent.
- Normal developmental behaviours can also resemble PA. Healthy adolescent autonomy is believed to be cultivated when parents support their children to develop relationships independently of them. A desire to spend more time with friends and less with parents can be healthy and does not necessarily reflect a poor relationship with a parent. Criticisms of a parent by an adolescent can also be present, but constant harsh attacks on a parent suggest further investigation is required to try to establish whether this is within an average range of behaviours.

Justifiable estrangement

Justifiable estrangement describes a situation whereby a child rejects a parent for an appropriate reason. Reasons for estrangement can include betrayal, poor parenting and abuse, with major issues associated with lack of trust and emotional closeness (13). One study interviewed 25 adults who did not have contact with their parents, and although they said they terminated contact so that they could heal from the impact of the relationship, they also described feeling loss for many years (14). Despite this, most did not miss their estranged parent and did not want to change their situation. However, it appeared that the estrangement impacted on their other relationships including partners, work colleagues and friends.

Some parents feel there is never a justifiable reason for estrangement, and parents can have high expectations for their children, even if they have not necessarily behaved reasonably towards them. However, if a parent is abusive, disrespectful or violent and/or has a drug/alcohol issue or a severe and enduring mental illness that means they do not have the capacity to engage in parenting at times, then it is reasonable for a child to want to withdraw emotionally. If the last memory a child has of their estranged parent is of them staggering into their home and hitting them or others or behaving in a threatening manner, then it is reasonable that they will be averse to further contact. If they no longer have to spend time with a parent they perceive as a threat, then they might be relieved; they are able to engage with their lives without having to worry about whether the estranged parent will behave reasonably. Many children say they do not want to see parents who leave them in their extended family's home, e.g. with grandparents, aunts and uncles, then go and do other things, although this is also something that is said by alienated children and highlights the need to consider all the information available during assessment. Children of parents with substance use disorders described feeling concerned about their parents even if they did not see them, and it seemed that there were some conflicting and contradictory emotions experienced (15).

Some experienced evaluators report that it can be helpful to try to establish when the estrangement began to emerge and consider all the possible explanations, rather than jump to conclusions (2). For example, there may be PA, but then again, there are occasions when a child's personality begins to develop and simply does not 'fit' with the adult's personality, and this results in a clash any time they meet. In this situation a struggle between the personalities might have been present before any parental separation. Therefore, if the child does not want to see the nonpreferred parent after separation and there is a history of a poor relationship, the child's decision might be made entirely independently of the preferred parent. It has also been noted that there are occasions when a past good relationship could 'derail' during a parental separation, which means that past positive exchanges are not concrete evidence that the relationship had not deteriorated before or during the period when the nonpreferred parent moved out (2).

Allegations of domestic violence

The negative impact of domestic violence on children is well established (16), and alienating parents often allege that they do not want their child to have contact with the targeted parent because they have a history of violence, raising issues of concern from professionals involved. Typically, alienating parents say that the violence was present throughout the relationship, although they sometimes describe one or two incidents. They often say they remained in the relationship because they loved their partner, thought they would change or were too frightened to leave. If they did not contact the police, they often say this was because they were too frightened to call them. There is variability in a situation where domestic violence is alleged, and sometimes the police have been called out to the homes of targeted parents accused of domestic violence. Some targeted parents say that the alienating parent deliberately phoned the police, knowing that the call would be recorded. They claim they were not aggressive and simply turned up at an agreed time or met them in the street. Sometimes they say they did not even speak to the alienating parent, and there are occasions when it is hard for professionals to know whom to believe. This supports the need for a thorough assessment of the family and their situation.

When the targeted parent is asked about allegations of violence, they often accuse the alienating parent of being the violent one, and so professionals reach another impasse in these incredibly complex cases. Police reports can be used as supporting information at times, but when law enforcement was not contacted, professionals are left with only their opinion about the likelihood of violence. An assessment of the targeted parent's history is necessary, and any tendency towards violence is recorded and commented on. When it is alleged that the targeted parent was violent, this is then often used as a reason to prevent contact from taking place. Sometimes this is supported by 'evidence' from newspaper stories depicting children who have been hurt by their parents during contact. The alienating parent often does not accept the opinion of the expert on whether their ex-partner is likely to be violent or not.

Sometimes a targeted parent has to cope with allegations of violence where none has taken place, but the alienating parent has been violent towards them. This is not easy for anyone who has experienced this situation, and sometimes it can make the targeted parent angry, but when they present with high arousal, this provides 'evidence' for the alienating parent's allegations. Some parents remain calm in the face of numerous dishonest allegations made against them and manage to treat these as part of their process.

If the nonpreferred parent has been violent to the preferred parent during their relationship, then this raises other issues. In addition, the nonpreferred parent might be conflictual with a child during contact. Some studies have found that children will often remain in a conflictual relationship with a parent, even if they are abusive (17), and the focus of the assessment has to be on protecting the child and thinking about what is best for them.

The frequency with which the alienating parent alleges violence and how this poses a risk to the child raises the issue of assessing for violence potential, causing anxiety for any expert/professional involved, and should form part of any assessment.

Child-motivated alienation

There are occasions when a child does not have a positive relationship with one parent, sometimes because of their experiences during the parental separation and sometimes because they simply did not have a good history with them. If they had a positive relationship in the past but the situation changed during the breakdown of the parents' relationship, then it has been reported that this can impact on the likelihood of the child enjoying a potentially rewarding relationship with their nonpreferred parent as a result of a temporary situation (2). In this situation, the favoured parent can contribute to any reduction in affection by denigrating the non-preferred parent, or they can behave in a laissez-faire fashion and fail to support the child to make a choice to see their other parent. This can then result in estrangement.

It is believed that cases of child-driven alienation do not occur very often, and it is therefore important that the court assessor considers the behaviour of the preferred parent during the relationship breakdown (2). The difficulty is that often when the preferred parent is trying to adjust to a relationship ending, it can be hard to convince them that their child needs their other parent, too. For this reason, adjustment time is particularly important for the preferred parent.

Conclusion

Assessments in cases of PA can be extremely complex and the behaviours difficult to identify and describe conclusively. There are occasions when estrangement appears to be justified and the targeted parent has contributed to their situation, and also, there are times when the child has reasonable as well as unreasonable thoughts about their nonpreferred parent. Their conflict can be supported by the preferred parent, or they might take a laissez-faire approach and not attempt to support the child to change their thinking. The harm that this might cause the child does not appear to be prioritised, or it might not be recognised or considered a serious issue. If the child wants to support their preferred parent, they might not tell them just how much pressure the situation places them under.

The onus is on the court expert to ensure that all potential explanations for a child's behaviour are considered and discussed before deciding that a preferred parent has shown alienating behaviours. Court experts have to provide evidence to support their assertions with information gathered during the assessment and be convincing when they present their conclusions. This means that an emphasis on appropriate expert witness training or knowledge is required before any court expert undertakes a case of this complexity. Education and training regarding the complexity of alienating behaviours and exceptions to this are critical.

References

1   Warshak, R.A. (2015). Ten parental alienation fallacies that compromise decisions in court and in therapy. *Professional Psychology: Research and Practice*, 46, 235–249. doi:10.1037/pro0000031.
2   Warshak, R.A. (2019). When evaluators get it wrong: False positives IDs and parental alienation. *Psychology, Public Policy and Law*, 26, 54–68. doi:10.1037/law0000216.
3   Bala, N., Hunt, S. and McCarney, C. (2010). Parental alienation: Canadian court cases 1989–2008. *Family Court Review*, 48, 164–179. doi:10.1111/j.1744-1617.2009.01269.x.
4   Gardner, R.S. (2002). Denial of the parental alienation syndrome also harms women. *American Journal of Family Therapy*, 30, 191–202. doi:10.1080/019261802753577520.
5   Kopetski, L.M., Rand, D.C. and Rand, R. (2006). Incident, gender and false allegations of child abuse: Data on 84 parental alienation syndrome cases. In R.S. Gardner, D.S. Sauber and D. Lorandos (Eds.), *The international handbook of parental alienation syndrome: Conceptual, clinical and legal considerations* (pp. 65–70). Springfield, IL: Charles C. Thomas Publisher.
6   Warshak, R.A. (2010). *Divorce poison: How to protect your family from bad-mouthing and brainwashing*. New York: HarperCollins.
7   Fidler, B.J., Bala, N., Birnbaum, R. and Kavassalis, K. (2008). *Challenging issues in child custody disputes*. Ontario, Canada: Carswell.

 8 Weir, K. (2011). High conflict contact disputes: Evidence of the extreme unreliability of some children's ascertainable wishes and feelings. *Family Court Review*, 49, 788–800. doi:10.1111/j.1744-1617.2011.01414.x.

 9 Garber, B.D. (2015). Cognitive-behavioural methods in high-conflict divorce: Systematic desensitization adapted to parent-child reunification interventions. *Family Court Review*, 53, 96–112. doi:10.1111/fcre.12133.

10 Weir, K. and Sturge, C. (2006). Clinical advice to courts on children's contact with their parents following parental separation. *Child and Adolescent Mental Health*, 11, 40–46. doi:10.1111/j.1475-3588.2005.00385_1.x.

11 Baker, A.J.L. (2005). The long-term effects of parental alienation on adult children: A qualitative research study. *American Journal of Family Therapy*, 33, 289–302. doi:10.1080/01926180590962129.

12 Friedlander, S. and Walters, M.G. (2010). When a child rejects a parent: Tailoring the intervention to fit the problem. *Family Court Review*, 48, 98–111. doi:10.1111/j.1744-1617.2009.01291.x.

13 Linden, A.H. and Sillence, E. (2021). "I'm finally allowed to be me": Parent-child estrangement and psychological wellbeing. *Families Relationships and Societies*, 10, 325–241. doi:10.1332/204674319X15647593365505.

14 Agllias, K. (2017). Missing family: The adult child's experience of parental estrangement. *Journal of Social Work Practice*, 32, 59–72. doi:10.1080/02650533.2017.1326471.

15 Wangensteen, T., Bramness, J.G. and Halsa, A. (2018). Growing up with parental substance use disorder: The struggle with complex emotions, regulation of contact, and lack of professional support. *Child and Family Social Work*, 24, 201–208. doi:10.1111/cfs.12603.

16 Holt, S. (2016). 'Quality' contact post separation/divorce: A review of the literature. *Child and Youth Services Review*, 68, 92–99. doi:10.1016/j.childyouth.2016.07.001.

17 Block, S.D., Oran, H., Oran, D., Baumrind, N. and Goodman, G.S. (2010). Abused and neglected children in court: Knowledge and attitudes. *Child Abuse and Neglect*, 34, 659–670. doi:10.1016/j.chiabu.2010.02.003.

Chapter 5

The alienating parent

Introduction

In the UK, all mothers and the majority of fathers have legal rights and responsibilities, known as 'parental responsibility'. If a parent has 'parental responsibility' this means they are expected to provide a home for their child and protect and maintain the child. They have a say in their education, medical treatment, how they are disciplined and how the child's property is to be looked after. They are also required to give permission for a change of name. This means that even if a parent with parental responsibility does not live with the family, the other parent must consider their views when making significant decisions about the welfare of the child (1). Mothers automatically have parental responsibility, and fathers have it if they are married to the mother or named on the birth certificate. If not, they can apply for it and either obtain the mother's agreement or a court order to give them parental responsibility. Same-sex parents have parental responsibility if they are both the child's legal parents. The term 'parental responsibility' emphasises the importance of the role for those who hold it. Sadly, in cases of parental alienation the child's needs are not typically the priority. Some parents fail to meet the requirements associated with parental responsibility, and often alienating parents ignore or minimise their duties. This requires the targeted parent to employ legal representation to try to have their rights enforced by the court. It is the law that children should have contact with both parents, and when the child does not live with one parent, the resident parent must ensure that the child's needs are met by supporting them to see the non-resident parent.

After separation the parents need to be able to establish a workable relationship and ensure the child's welfare is the priority. The roles will change, and the non-resident parent may find it difficult to define their position at first. In one study of resident parents who were mothers, it was found that there was less conflict between parents when mothers were happy with their divorce settlement and perceived the father's role positively. It seemed that mothers who experienced the highest levels of stress were most likely to have conflictual relationships with the fathers, and this raises the importance of support for separating parents during the period of adjustment that typically follows separation (2).

DOI: 10.4324/9781003156147-5

In cases where alienation is thought to occur, the resident parent is usually believed to be manipulating the child. As a result of the manipulation, the child says they no longer want a relationship with the targeted parent. The goal of the alienating parent is therefore to try to stop the relationship between the child and the targeted parent and also usually their extended family, or in milder cases they wish to control these relationships and minimise their relevance or importance for the child. The alienating parent is most frequently the mother, but it can also be the father. It has been noted that the alienating parent's close family members are often also involved in the alienation process, and sometimes the alienating parent has the support of their extended family, such as grandparents or aunts or uncles (3).

Sometimes the resident and alienating parent is very transparent, and whilst giving frivolous excuses for the child not wanting to see their other parent, they flaunt their perceived control. At times they present as very sincere and concerned about the child, and sometimes they may be dramatic and cry, claiming that the courts are trying to reunite the child with a dangerous or neglectful parent, when (they say) the child has clearly stated they do not want to go to contact. Some parents rapidly switch from charming to verbally aggressive in seconds and then back again to a calm presentation if they are appeased. Because of the disparate presentations of alienating parents, it can be difficult to try to remain balanced when working with parental alienation cases. There is no doubt it is stressful for professionals trying to help the situation, and in addition, alienating parents are often quick to criticise and can make insulting or personal remarks about those who do not automatically side with them.

To bring some compassion to the situation, it is important to remember that whilst we may all have had different experiences in life, we also have a lot in common. Each individual who gets involved in protracted proceedings had a history from which they learned coping strategies and interaction styles. The alienating parent may hold a particular point of view because of their life experiences. In addition, some people struggle to understand that others may hold a different opinion from themselves. An alienating parent might lack empathy for others or their children, and this may not be due to negligence or a deliberate act by them but rather a personality characteristic and resistance to change. They may be sensitive to criticism, leading to feelings of distress, anger and defensiveness, particularly if they feel threatened. It is also the case that most alienating parents appear to have experienced some disturbance in their own family life by way of conflict, although many do not acknowledge it and the history comes from other sources. It seems this disturbance in their own history, which might not be recognised by them, has increased the likelihood of alienating parents often presenting themselves poorly, as described above. This is consistent with reports that there can be significant conflict within the family of origin of alienating parents, even though they may describe their history in an idealistic fashion (4).

Obviously, no-one is at their best during a relationship breakdown, which is a process and usually involves a period of grieving or adjustment whilst at the same time the relationship is ending. During the adjustment process people may experience despair, sadness, loss and anger. These emotional experiences can influence how they perceive their departing partner and also how they behave. The person who is leaving the relationship may leave behind someone who is angry and alone and who uses the child for emotional support, sometimes because they do not have anyone else and therefore they feel they need the child to be 'on their side' as they see it, and they do not free the child up or give them permission to have a relationship with the other parent.

Some alienating parents talk about revenge on the targeted parent, and this can reflect how hurt they feel, although it indicates they have lost sight of the impact of their behaviours on their child. Others have a new life, partner and/or child, and they no longer need the targeted parent. They appear to feel that with a new partner, things would be less complicated if they could just forget about their ex-partner and encourage the child to engage with their new 'mum' or 'dad'. Of course, if this next relationship does not last, then it can be very complicated for the child, who might have to manage loss again. Psychoeducation about this situation is unhelpful, since at the beginning of a relationship, people tend to feel positive about their future and are not thinking about the possibility of an ending.

Problems with the literature

There is a significant challenge involved in collecting information from participants who do not wish to admit to alienating behaviours, and this presents a problem for those attempting to study this group of individuals. Typically, alienating parents do not acknowledge any weakness or limitations, and they do not engage with professionals, even if it appears that they do. It is also unlikely that an alienating parent would admit to covert behaviours, such as giving misleading information to the alienated child or their targeted parent. A small number of alienating parents when the truth emerges will admit that they 'made it all up', although this is not usual.

Due to the difficulties with reliable data collection from alienating parents, many of the research studies looking at this situation have considered the narrative of the child in retrospect by asking for the opinion of college/university students, or they have gathered information from the targeted parent, whilst others have used information from the courts (5–7). This is all valuable data since it gives an account of the experience of other people involved with the alienating parent.

Goal of the alienating parent

The goal of the alienating parent is to remove the targeted parent from the child's life or minimise their role as a parent. In the home of an alienating parent, there is often an absence of pictures of the child's 'other' family, and sometimes there are numerous pictures of the alienating parent's family. Attempts to draw attention to this are dismissed and minimised. It is understandable that an alienating parent might not want to look at pictures of their ex-partner, particularly if the separation was acrimonious; however, as the ex-partner continues to be their child's parent and will (hopefully) remain in their lives, there is an extent to which the alienating parent is required to tolerate their ex-partner for the benefit of their child. In other words, like all good parents, they need to be able to prioritise the child's need to have a relationship with the other parent, above any feelings they have about not wanting their ex-partner around.

Causes and motivations of the alienating parent

There are many reasons for alienating behaviours, such as wanting to be the preferred parent or avoiding alone time, and some clinicians feel a dominant motivator for alienating parents is revenge (8). Others report that a combination of anger and pathology led to parents having problems separating from their child and recognising social boundaries (9). Overall, the thinking from researchers to date has been around the alienating parent having personality issues, such as high dependency needs, narcissism or boundary issues, in addition to fears of abandonment, feelings of anger and revenge, or emotional/mental health difficulties.

Some authors have considered whether the alienating parent's issues relate to a problem with interpersonal boundaries, and three ways have been proposed whereby an alienating parent's relationship with their child may impact on contact with the targeted parent (10). Firstly, a child may become 'parentified' so that they want to care for the main adult in their lives, who may be alone after the targeted parent leaves home. Next, the child might become a peer or partner for the alienating parent, and in this way, the child is the alienating parent's friend and confidante, which is known as 'adultified'. Finally, the parent 'infantilises' the child, so that they are not encouraged to develop in the same way as their peer group but rather remain close to the alienating parent. These suggestions appear to be consistent with the thoughts of other clinicians about a parent not wanting to be alone (8) and also observations about the alienating parent's social boundaries with the child (9).

In many situations the alienating parent has a new partner, and it appears the ex-partner has been cast aside as though they are no longer required. The alienating parent does not appear to consider the impact on the child of switching parents or adding in new siblings, to perhaps remove or replace them again later. There is a lack of acknowledgement of the child's needs or empathy for their situation. There is also a problem with boundaries, as the child's needs are ignored and their relationship with their other parent is not protected, as it needs to be.

There are some aspects of the alienating parent's functioning that are understandable – not always reasonable, but understandable. For example, they may see their ex-partner presenting as happy and apparently leading a good life, whilst they may feel alone and unhappy and embittered. Some authors have reported that this can 'serve as a lightning rod for rage' (9). This happens if the alienating parent feels the ex-partner mistreated them yet has gone on to be happy and fulfilled, and they may feel there has been an injustice. For some individuals this results in feelings of victimisation, and for others it leads to thoughts about revenge. A small number of parents (mothers) have eventually told me that they lied about their ex-partners sexually assaulting their children, and that this was associated with 'revenge'. The parents who described this were insightful even if they were not remorseful. On reflection, they were able to recognise the reasoning for their behaviours, although not all alienating parents are able to do this.

In a study of the views of eight psychologists working with PA in South Africa there have been findings that the problems were becoming more prevalent (11). It was considered PA was associated with people in relationships 'decoupling' at different times, so that one person was happy with the separation but the other felt left behind. This makes sense, since if one person remains invested in the relationship whilst the other person is planning to leave, it could lead to the individual left behind feeling abandoned. It was considered that some parents might act unconsciously. The parents are so distraught with their situation that they act irrationally, and the child is caught up in the process. In the alienating parent's mind, the child might be harmed by the targeted parent despite the lack of evidence to suggest this is the case. The authors in this study noted that working with alienating parents was difficult because 'you don't find logic, reasoning or solutions', and like other authors, they noted that alienating parents were not acting in the best interests of their child but rather were focused on their own goals (11).

Others also noted the issues relating to abandonment and associated with feelings of rejection and humiliation. One of the reasons for alienation that has been suggested is an abnormal grief reaction to the relationship ending (4). The alienating parent does not want the relationship to end, and so it continues in conflict through the courts. The alienating parent does not attempt to maintain the relationship through the child, as feelings of anger and hostility lead them to want to hurt the other parent, who did not remain in the relationship.

One study examined 16 alienating parents and found they all had feelings of sadness which they blamed on their ex-partner (12). It has been suggested that blaming the other parent is important since it means the alienating parent avoids facing responsibility for any problems they encounter (4) and that the alienating parent wishes to be in control, and when the relationship does not proceed as they planned, they are then looking for revenge. This is consistent with the interpretation of the behaviour by others who felt that alienating parents turned their emotional pain into conflict (13). Therefore, a number of theories have been proposed to explain why one parent alienates a child against another parent. These are considered in more detail in the following pages.

Revenge and anger

Revenge and anger are frequently referred to in the PA literature and during clinical evaluation. Revenge is a behaviour that results sometimes when someone perceives a wrongdoing towards them by another. It is intended to cause harm to the other person involved and can be an action or the withdrawal of something that the other person wants. It is typically an aggressive act. Studies have shown that revenge is typically about retribution rather than an effort to deter future harm (14). The individual who wants to invoke revenge feels it unfair that the other party appears happy whilst they feel sad and hurt. This unhappiness, if admitted by an alienating parent, could be a focus for intervention in PA cases. The research shows that people seek révenge to try to improve hurt feelings, and revenge fantasies are emotionally satisfying (15). There are findings that anger, contempt, jealousy and envy may cause revenge (16), and people with 'just world beliefs' (they believe in a 'just' world) are more likely to seek vengeance for perceived misdoings than others (17). Thoughts about revenge are likely to be associated with the level of injustice that is believed to have occurred (18), with revenge seekers believing that for justice to be done, the magnitude of revenge should be greater than the original harm incurred (19). Some people seek revenge even when it offers no obvious benefit (14). It has been reported that there is a logic to revenge, and it can be functional, i.e. serve a purpose. If the transgression against someone is perceived as intentional, then this is typically judged as a greater injustice than an unintentional act (20). Anger plays a significant role in revenge, and those with personality types that are characterised by anger, such as narcissistic personalities, are more likely to seek revenge (21). People who are strongly narcissistic are more likely than others to exact revenge when they feel they have been disrespected, and this is because they feel they deserve special attention from others (21). This is consistent with reports that narcissistic personality characteristics are prevalent in alienating parents (22).

Some alienating parents have admitted they alienated their child out of 'revenge', and there are findings that an apology can reduce the need for vengeance (23). It is believed this is because it alleviates concern about future offences and restores a sense of balance, and the individual involved feels respected. There are also findings that people who feel chronically powerless and find themselves in a position of power may abuse this through revenge, whereas people who usually have power in their lives do not have the same drives (24). People are less likely to take revenge if they feel their opponent is more powerful than they are (25), and it has been found that goals for revenge can be to make the other person suffer but also can involve improving a relationship through regulation, repair or strengthening (26). Motivations for revenge can depend on the context of the relationship, and there has been very little research examining the underpinnings of revenge in interpersonal relationships. It has been found that people perceive others as engaging in vengeful acts more frequently than themselves, and when asked, people incorrectly considered it likely that acts of revenge would be perceived positively by others. It was felt there was a social norm and expectation for revenge in particular circumstances (26). This is consistent with PA, as some alienating parents have reported their decision to intervene in the relationship between a child and a parent is an act of revenge.

Problems with boundaries

Sometimes it appears to be the case that the alienating parent feels that they love the child so much that they cannot share them; however, if they do this, then they are prioritising their own needs above those of the child. The alienating parent may have high dependency needs (they are highly dependent on others), which supports theories relating to parentification/adultification, or the alienating parent may be frightened of losing the child to the targeted parent (10). I remember once a nursery schoolteacher telling me a particular parent was in the nursery every day, even though the child did not need them there. She said, 'the mother's needs are greater than the child's' or words to that effect, and sometimes in alienation cases, it may be the case that the carer's child fulfils the carer's own personal needs, and they cannot possibly permit anyone else to get close to the child, particularly an ex-partner. The alienating parent may not always be aware of using the child to try to fulfil their own needs and may perceive themselves as 'caring'.

The alienating parent's awareness of the impact on the child

There are no specific studies that I could identify that considered the alienating parent's thoughts about the impact of alienation on the child. In my experience, if someone tries to explain to the alienating parent that they are harming their child, they appear not to listen, or perhaps they do not believe the professional, or they might not care. It might be the case that there are different reasons for alienation and that some parents might not be aware they are doing this. It is also possible alienating parents lack empathy for their child and the targeted parent. On many occasions when alienating parents present as virtuous, I indicate to them the benefits of child/absent parent contact and wonder whether it might be unkind to stop their child seeing the targeted parent without good reason. The alienating parent typically dismisses this idea or ignores it. Empathy is a concept that alienating parents seem to struggle with, and the impact of their behaviours on their child is not something they appear to be concerned about. More frequently they say the child will be harmed by seeing the targeted parent.

When the other parent has left, the primary caregiver may feel aggrieved because they have been left, as they see it, with the responsibility and work associated with childcare and often with reduced financial income. Meanwhile, the person who has left the family home may feel the primary caregiver is controlling and obstructive. Often both parents feel that the other parent is being difficult, and this results in an increase in irrational behaviour, particularly if the parents are experiencing their own emotional turmoil as a result of the separation. For a child living with their primary caregiver, this may be the beginning, or continuation, of a gradual erosion of the relationship with the non-resident parent, that is, if the resident parent decides to alienate the child from the targeted parent.

Other findings about personality characteristics

It seems there is not one particular personality type who is likely to alienate their child against an ex-partner, although some personality traits are over-represented (22). There has been some discussion about whether alienating parents may have some disturbance in personality that leads to a tendency to be manipulative, as well as having difficulty separating their needs from those of the child, and they may struggle to communicate information in a forthright manner (27).

One study in the US compared two groups of parents on a formal measure of personality, the MMPI-2 (Minnesota Multiphasic Personality Inventory – 2nd edition), and categorised the groups as alienating or not, based on the child custody evaluator's account of their behaviours (28). Sixteen parents were deemed to be alienating, and 18 were not. The researchers found the alienating group were more likely to be defensive and presented themselves favourably. They tended to present themselves as highly virtuous and without any emotional problems or difficulties. Similarly, an Italian study analysed the personality profile of 81 mothers involved in child custody disputes (29). After exclusions they had 41 alienating mothers and 40 non-alienating mothers from four custody evaluators. The mothers were formally assessed, also using the MMPI-2. The researchers found that mothers who alienated children were more extroverted and felt they were more moral and virtuous than the other, non-alienating parents. In addition, they were more vulnerable to the impact of stress and had difficulty representing themselves. They perceived themselves favourably and lacked insight into their own frailties. Associated with this, they tended to deny problems and weaknesses and presented themselves in a way that was inconsistent with real life. It was also noted that alienating mothers were self-focused and predictable, demonstrated stereotypical viewpoints and were narrow-minded and naïve. They were reluctant to change and vulnerable to stress, although they attempted to deny the impact of distress by under-reporting their issues. The alienating parents also proclaimed more confidence in social situations and felt they contained their emotions when they were stressed. They indicated they did not experience social anxiety or embarrassment and said they abhorred violence. It was noted that the alienating mothers' perceptions of themselves were quite different from the view of others, who typically saw them as self-focused, predictable and unoriginal; having stereotyped thinking; and being narrow-minded, naïve and inflexible in their outlook on life. They were perceived as tending to be slow to adjust to new situations and particularly vulnerable to stress. It was felt that alienating mothers attempted to appear conventional and, in doing so, denied any distress, alienation or abnormality, which meant they minimised problems much more than non-alienating mothers (29).

Parents who present with the types of behaviours described as alienating want others to pay attention to what they say. They are manipulative and persuasive and stress that their ex-partner is the one to be wary of. They use their personality characteristics to place emotional pressure on professionals to write what they think, and the aim is to disrupt the relationship between their child and the other targeted parent. They often describe the targeted parent as manipulative and potentially dangerous. If the professional does not meet the targeted parent, they may assume that what the alienating parent says is correct, and they can be used by the alienating parent to hurt the targeted parent. It is possible that the alienating parent may not always be fully aware of their behaviours, but rather in the midst of the chaos that takes place around a relationship ending, they inadvertently include the children in their efforts to hurt the other parent. One of my colleagues said, 'when you told me about parental alienation, I wondered if I'd alienated my child, but when I really thought about it, I knew that I hadn't done'. The difference between my colleague and an alienating parent is that they reflected on their behaviours, and they knew that no matter how angry they had been when their relationship ended and even if they had been thinking about revenge, they had not hurt their child by including them in their relationship break-up.

Alienating parents often ignore professional advice, which can be offered due to court or social services intervention. When they try to use professionals to support their arguments, they give information that they believe will support their case. Frequently, this involves accusing the ex-partner of violence and suggesting that by permitting the child contact with the absent parent, the child will be emotionally or physically harmed or sexually assaulted. The alienating parent can shout, cry or sometimes present as vulnerable, and if challenged, a typical comment might be 'you're making me feel uncomfortable/bad/sad, etc.'. This is an example of manipulation and a strategy to get the evaluator to stop asking them questions. The behaviour will be transparent to an experienced assessor, but court experts, like all people, can sometimes be manipulated by alienating parents, who are sometimes very skilled. It is frequently the case that the alienating parents will make the professional feel uncomfortable by either raising their voice or presenting as helpless and putting the expert into a position whereby they feel they cannot continue without causing harm.

There are some reports that alienating parents were sometimes abusive partners before their relationship with the targeted parent ended, and PA is therefore a continuation of the abuse (30). The tendency of the alienating parent to be manipulative is a feature of the personality that can sometimes contribute to the relationship ending (4). One study found that parents who felt a lack of control during a relationship separation were more likely to make inappropriate disclosures about their separation process to their children (31). When they did, this sometimes had a negative effect on any child involved and was stressful for them. Although these parents were not all involved in PA, it highlights the need for parental supports during separation if the child's needs are to be protected.

Pathology of the alienating parent

The alienating parent typically presents as highly anxious about the child's welfare. They might be highly anxious about the child, particularly if they see them as an extension of themselves, although this leads us back to issues with boundaries.

They express concern about the targeted parent harming the child. Alternatively, the alienating parent may say this to justify their own unreasonable behaviour. Alienating parents say, 'they don't want to go' (to meet the targeted parent), or they say the targeted parent is violent or going to 'kill' the child. They sometimes say, 'they hurt me, so how do I know they won't hurt the child?', and if there has been domestic violence (or even allegations of aggression) in the relationship, then parents use this as 'evidence' that the absent parent may hurt their children. Sometimes alienating parents accuse targeted parents of aggression when it is not true, as a way of justifying their behaviours.

Emotional impact on the alienating parent

In relation to supporting the emotional wellbeing of the alienating parent, it has been noted that good intimate partner relationships have a positive impact on emotional welfare (32). Other characteristics have a negative impact on emotional welfare, and these are difficulty with emotional regulation, blaming the other partner and a refusal to communicate or cooperate. Even after separation a conflictual relationship is unlikely to be helpful to the alienating parent. There is likely to be a level of stress associated with engaging in PA, for example, visiting professionals to discuss the latest allegation, brooding about the outcomes, working out what to say next, trying to remember what they told the last professional if they were not forthright, etc. Studies looking at co-parenting and support after parental separation found that a resident mother's satisfaction with the separation agreement, perception of the father's ability to parent effectively, together with their having a positive view of the role of the father in the child's life, all predicted less stress in the resident mother (2). In support of this there are findings that alienating parents are more vulnerable to stress; therefore they need support, even if they are resistant when others attempt to help them (29).

There is significant research to show that poor relationships have a negative impact on emotional welfare, with findings that separation, conflict, problems and arguments all increase the likelihood of suicidality (33). If parents who carry out alienating behaviours struggle with the emotional impact of the separation, then this is likely to impact on their children, and there is significant evidence considering the impact of parental mental health and behaviours on their children (34). Children of parents with mental health problems are significantly more likely than their peer group to have emotional disturbances, and there are findings that in parents of children with mental health problems, 36% of mothers and 33% of fathers have similar issues (35).

Gender issues

There have been comments that women's rights activists and others who deny alienation based on the premise that it is abusive towards women are ignoring the fact that many women are alienated from their children by men, and so they do a great disservice to them and their children (36).

It has been reported that in a study of the number of PA cases in lower and higher courts in the US between 1985 and 2018, 75% of the alienators were women and 25% were men (6). Despite the many males who alienated and the fact that there are women who suffer greatly due to this behaviour, there are reports that allegations of PA are insulting to women. This is because of the many alienating parents who are mothers (29). However, it has been pointed out that it is often females who have children in their care after separation, and given that the alienating parent is typically the resident parent, it makes sense that more females will be alienating parents than males (37). Similarly, early studies showed that mothers were more likely to alienate their children than fathers, with findings that when litigation was involved, children were much more likely to align themselves with the mother than the father (38).

More recently, in Canada it was found that mothers were more than twice as likely to be accused of PA than fathers; however, allegations against fathers were more likely to be accepted in the court (39). Overall, findings of alienation were most likely to be made against parents with sole custody who were mostly mothers, and in 48% of cases, the residence arrangement was changed to the targeted parent. There are findings that the resident parent is most likely to be the alienating parent and also that being the custodial parent does not cause PA but rather facilitates it (40–41). There are occasions when the non-resident parent alienates the child against the resident parent, although these cases are seen less often.

One study considered how mothers and fathers perceived their parenting roles and whether alienating behaviours were more acceptable if they were carried out by a mother (42). Although the researchers found that alienating behaviours were generally perceived negatively, they also found that behaviour which aimed to improve loyalty to one parent whilst portraying the other parent negatively and attempts to reduce the salience of the relationship with the targeted parent were considered more favourably when carried out by the mother. They believed that this was because mothers were often perceived as being 'protective', and their behaviour was considered justifiable considering that fathers sometimes behaved poorly. Their data also suggested that fathers were more likely to be rewarded for 'normal' parenting behaviour than mothers, who were expected to be positive parents.

Although one study found no difference in the strategies used by different genders (43), there are also findings that there are gender differences in the way parents use alienation and reports that mothers are more likely to use indirect methods, such as denigrating the targeted parent and filing many false allegations of abuse against the targeted parent (44). However, the researchers did not find that alienating fathers were more aggressive than mothers, but in fact fathers used the same methods (women used more of them), and the researchers discussed whether this was because direct aggression was much more obvious than indirect.

There are other findings of gender differences in the types of alienation displayed by parents (41, 45) and it has been noted that mothers who alienate are more likely to engage their new partner to fulfil a parenting role, seek medical/psychological reports as evidence to support their assertions and/or seek accomplices for alienating (41). Men, on the other hand, were more likely to encourage the child to challenge or defy the targeted parent. It was reported that mothers were significantly more likely than fathers to be on the receiving end of denigration tactics and was suggested that males may take a more aggressive approach to reduce a targeted mother's hold over their child (45). Other studies have found that both mothers and fathers were equally likely to engage in alienating behaviours (5), and some investigations which have not focused on PA have found that during divorce there is no gender difference in Machiavellianism (41, 46).

Conclusion

Alienating behaviours occur for a variety of reasons, and both aspects of personality and the emotional wellbeing of the alienating parent motivate them to behave in a particular manner. From the research, revenge and anger, difficulty with boundaries and problems with adjusting to the end of the relationship appear to be motivations for PA. It is clear that some personalities are more likely to alienate than others, and a tendency to be narcissistic with feelings of moral superiority has been reported. In addition, there are findings that extroverted mothers are more likely to engage in PA. There is also a tendency for alienating parents to be vulnerable to stress. There appears to be no gender difference in a parent's propensity to engage in PA. The rights and needs of the child are overlooked when alienation takes place, and alienating parents prioritise their own needs. In this way they have difficulty with boundaries and fail to recognise their responsibilities as a parent.

In terms of future research, one research group noted it would be helpful to know whether there might be alienating parent personality characteristics that protect a child from the impact of PA, and similarly an area for exploration might be whether some features of the child are helpful, such as resilience and high self-esteem (29). This is particularly important since, consistent with other experts, these authors note that *'once on the road to alienation, parents are not likely to stop on their own accord'* (29, p. 16).

References

1 UK Government Website. (2021). www.gov.uk/parental-rights-responsibilities (Accessed 14 September 2021).
2 Petren, R.E., Ferraro, A.J., Davis, T.R. and Pasley, K. (2017). Factors linked with coparenting support and conflict after divorce. *Journal of Divorce and Remarriage*, 58. doi:10.1080/10502556.2017.1300013.
3 Vassiliou, D. and Cartwright, G.F. (2001). The lost parents' perspective on parental alienation syndrome. *American Journal of Family Therapy*, 29, 181–191. doi:10.1080/019261801750424307.
4 Haines, J., Matthewson, M. and Turnbull, M. (2020). *Understanding and managing parental alienation: A guide to assessment and intervention.* Oxon: Routledge.

5 Hands, A.J. and Warshak, R.A. (2011). Parental alienation among college students. *The American Journal of Family Therapy*, 39, 431–443. http://dx.doi.org/10/1080/1092 6187.2011.

6 Lorandos, D. (2020). Parental alienation in US courts, 1985 to 2018. *Family Court Review*, 58, 322–339.

7 Maturana, S.L., Matthewson, M., Dwan, C. and Norris, K. (2018). Characteristics and experiences of targeted parents of parental alienation from their own perspective: A systematic literature review. *Australian Journal of Psychology*. doi:10.1111/ajpy.12226.

8 Gardner, R.A. (1998). *The parental alienation syndrome* (2nd edition). Cresskill, NJ: Creative Therapeutics Inc.

9 Kelly, J.B. and Johnston, J.R. (2001). The alienated child: A reformulation of parental alienation syndrome. *Family Court Review*, 39, 249–266.

10 Garber, B.A. (2011). Parental alienation and the dynamics of the enmeshed parent-child dyad: Adultification, parentification and infantilization. *Family Court Review*, 49, 322–335.

11 Viljoen, M. and van Rensburg, E. (2014). Exploring the lived experiences of psychologists working with parental alienation syndrome. *Journal of Divorce and Remarriage*, 55, 253–275. doi:10.1080/10502556.2014.901833.

12 Dunne, J. and Hedrick, M. (1994). The parental alienation syndrome: An analysis of sixteen selected cases. *Journal of Divorce and Remarriage*, 21, 21–38. doi:10.1300/J087v21n03_02.

13 Kopetski, L. (1998). Identifying cases of parental alienation syndrome – part II. *The Colorado Lawyer*, 27, 61–64.

14 Osgood, J.M. (2016). Is revenge about retributive justice, deterring harm, or both? *Social and Personality Psychology Compass*. doi:10.1111/spc3.12296.

15 Barber, L., Maltby, J. and Macaskill, A. (2005). Angry memories and thoughts of revenge: The relationship between forgiveness and anger rumination. *Personality and Individual Differences*, 39, 253–262.

16 Darley, J.M. and Pittman, T.S. (2003). The psychology of compensatory and retributive justice. *Personality and Social Psychology Review*, 40, 7, 324–336.

17 Ball, G.A., Trevino, L.K. and Sims, H.P. (1994). Just and unjust punishment: Influences on subordinate performance and citizenship. *Academy of Management Journal*, 37, 299–322.

18 Carlsmith, K.M. and Darley, J.M. (2008). Psychological aspects of retributive justice. *Advances in Experimental Social Psychology*, 40, 193–236.

19 Marongiu, P. and Newman, G. (1987). *Vengeance: The fight against injustice*. Totowa, NJ: Rowman and Littlefield.

20 Jackson, J.C., Choi, V.K. and Gelfant, M.J. (2019). Revenge: A multilevel review and synthesis. *Annual Review of Psychology*, 70, 319–345.

21 Rasmussen, K. (2016). Entitled vengeance: A meta-analysis relating narcissism to provoked aggression. *Aggressive Behavior*, 42, 362–379.

22 Baker, A.J.L. (2006). Patterns of parental alienation syndrome: A qualitative study of adults who were alienated from a parent as a child. *The American Journal of Family Therapy*, 34, 63–78. doi:10.1080/01926180500301444.

23 Govier, T. (2002). *Forgiveness and revenge*. New York: Psychology Press.

24 Azzam, T.I., Beaulieu, D.A. and Bugental, D.B. (2007). Anxiety and hostility to an 'outsider' as moderated by low perceived power. *Emotion*, 7, 660–667.

25 Aquino, K., Tripp, T.M. and Bies, R.J. (2006). Getting even or moving on. Power, procedural justice and types of offence as predictors of revenge, forgiveness, reconciliation and avoidance in organisations. *Journal of Applied Psychology*, 91, 653–668.

26 Boon, S.D. and Yoshimura, S.M. (2014). Pluralistic ignorance in revenge attitudes and behavior in interpersonal relationships. *Personal Relationships*. doi:10.1111/pere. 12030.

27 Baker, A. and Ben Ami, N. (2011). To turn a child against a parent is to turn a child against himself. *Journal of Divorce and Remarriage*, 54, 203–210. doi:10.1080/1050 2556.2011.609424.

28 Siegel, J.C. and Langford, J.S. (1998). MMPI-2 validity scales and suspected parental alienation syndrome. *American Journal of Forensic Psychology*, 16, 1–7.

29 Roma, P., Marchetti, D., Mazza, C., Burla, F. and Verrocchio, M.C. (2020). MMPI profiles of mothers engaged in parental alienation. *Journal of Family Issues*. doi:10.1177/0192513X20918393.

30 Harman, J.J., Kruk, E. and Hines, D. (2018). Parental alienating behaviors: An unacknowledged form of family violence. *Psychological Bulletin*, 144, 1275–1299. doi:10.1037/bul0000175.

31 Afifi, T.D., McManus, T., Hutchinson, S. and Baker, B. (2007). Inappropriate parental divorce disclosures, the factors that prompt them, and their impact on parents' and adolescents' well-being. *Communication Monographs*, 74. doi:10.1080/03637750701 196870.

32 Abela, A. (2020). The significance of the couple relationship in the twenty-first century. In A. Abela, S. Vella and S. Piscopo (Eds.), *Couple relationships in a global context. European family therapy association series*. Cham: Springer. doi:10.1007/978-3-030-37712-0_2.

33 Kazan, D., Calear, A.L. and Batterham, P.J. (2016). The impact of intimate partner relationships on suicidal thoughts and behaviours: A systematic review. *Journal of Affective Disorders*, 190, 585–598.

34 Albanese, A.M., Russo, G.R. and Geller, P.A. (2019). The role of parental self-efficacy in parent and child well-being: A systematic review of associated outcomes. *Child Care, Health and Development*, 45, 333–363. doi:10.1111/cch.12261.

35 Campbell, T.C.H., Reupert, A., Sutton, K., Basu, S., Davidson, G., Middeldorp, C.M., Naughton, M. and Maybery, D. (2021). Prevalence of mental illness among parents of children receiving treatment within child and adolescent mental health services (CAMHS): A scoping review. *European Child and Adolescent Psychiatry*, 30, 997–1012. doi:10.1007/s00787-020-01502-x.

36 Fidler, B.J. and Bala, N. (2010). Children resisting post-separation contact with a parent: Concepts, controversies and conundrums. *Family Court Review*, 48, 10–47.

37 Lowenstein, L.F. (2013). Is the concept of parental alienation a meaningful one? *Journal of Divorce and Remarriage*, 54, 658–667. doi:10.1080/10502556.2013.810980.

38 Johnston, J.R. (2003). Parental alignments and rejection: An empirical study of alienation in children of divorce. *Journal of the American Academy of Psychiatry and the Law*, 31, 158–170.

39 Sheehy, E. and Boyd, S.B. (2020). Penalizing women's fear: Intimate partner violence and parental alienation in Canadian child custody cases. *Journal of Social Welfare and Family Law*, 42, 80–91. doi:10.1080/09649069.2020.1701940.

40 Harman, J.J. and Biringen, Z. (2016). *Parents acting badly: How institutions and societies promote the alienation of children from their loving families*. Fort Collins: Colorado Parental Alienation Project, LLV.

41 López, T.J., Iglesias, V.E.N. and García, P.F. (2014). Parental alienation gradient: Strategies for a syndrome. *The American Journal of Family Therapy*, 42, 217–231. doi:10.1080/01926187.2013.820116.

42 Harman, J.J., Biringen, Z., Ratajack, E.M., Outland, P.L. and Kraus, A. (2016). Parents behaving badly: Gender biases in the perception of parental alienating behaviours. *Journal of Family Psychology*. doi:10.1037/fam0000232.

43 Baker, A.J.L. and Darnell, D. (2006). Behaviours and strategies employed in parental alienation: A survey of parental experiences. *Journal of Divorce and Remarriage*, 45, 97–124. doi:10.1300/J087v45n01_06.

44 Harman, J.J., Lorandos, D., Biringen, Z. and Grubb, C. (2019). Gender differences in the use of parental alienating behaviors. *Journal of Family Violence*. doi:10.1007/s10896-019-00097-5.

45 Balmer, S., Matthewson, M. and Haines, J. (2018). Parental alienation: Targeted parent perspective. *Australian Journal of Psychology*, 70, 91–99. doi:10.1111/ajpy.12159.

46 Clemente, M. and Diaz, Z. (2021). Machiavellianism and the manipulation of children as a tactic in child custody disputes: The MMS scale. *Journal of Forensic Psychology Research and Practice*, 21, 171–193. doi:10.1080/24732850.2020.1847525.

Chapter 6

The targeted parent

Introduction

Alienation is on a continuum, causing significant impairment in the lives of all involved, and as already discussed, some authors have applied a framework to this, referring to 'mild', 'moderate' and 'severe' parental alienation (1–2). Alienation can begin to occur at any stage of the parent/child relationship, and in some families, the targeted parent has been distanced from their child's life prior to the relationship ending. If one parent is preoccupied with meeting the child's needs, this could make the other parent feel ostracised and isolated, and whilst juggling relationship and childcare issues is demanding for anyone, a preoccupation with childcare can also be a symptom of dissatisfaction in the relationship. Therefore, if one parent is distracting themselves from problems by throwing themselves into other issues, it may either signify dissatisfaction or it can contribute to the relationship breakdown if either of the parents feels alone. Sadly, sometimes children become involved in a relationship þreakdown and strongly align themselves with one parent prior to the separation.

It may be difficult for a child and parent to develop their relationship after a separation if the connection was not strong when the parents were together, although for some children, the bond between them and their absent parent can develop later. This is because they are able to have uninterrupted time with their absent parent, who can focus on meeting their needs. They may develop shared interests as the child grows and the absent parent has an opportunity to enjoy aspects of their child's life without the mundane tasks of everyday life. This in itself can cause resentment and jealousy in a resident parent, and the journey is fraught with potential problems.

As mentioned earlier, parents are not usually 'at their best' during a separation, and feelings of anger, betrayal, disappointment and loss are prevalent. Often, both parents are sorry that a relationship has ended, no matter how complex the circumstances, and they need time to adjust to their new roles. When children are involved, the resident parent has to try to acclimatise quickly, so that they can provide a safe base for the children and address any behavioural or emotional

DOI: 10.4324/9781003156147-6

disturbance resulting from the break-up. The non-resident parent is required to try to negotiate with their ex-partner to agree on access times, work out how collections and drop-offs will be conducted, and communicate with professional bodies, such as school and medical providers. It can seem overwhelming for some parents.

There are occasions when the situation appears promising. Couples say that they are focused on supporting the children and therefore will not attempt to interfere with their relationships with others. Sometimes this works for a period; however, for many couples, the situation changes over time, particularly when another partner comes along, and the non-resident parent notices that children no longer want to meet them or spend time in their company. As we have already said, there are occasions when PA is identified when this is not the case; for example, a child refusing to attend contact occasionally is not in itself evidence of parental alienation, and although I have heard reports of professionals jumping to conclusions, most people working with these complex cases do their best to try to support individuals in this highly emotive and complicated situation. Targeted parents often start out with flexibility, and if the child involved has an apparently valid reason for missing contact, they simply re-arrange. There are of course exceptions to every situation, and some parents who later become targeted parents are complaining from the outset if their needs are not met.

The targeted parent usually intends to remain in their child's life after separating from the child's other parent. They usually hope to participate in the child's life, watch their sports activities, attend their school and extracurricular productions and parent-teacher meetings, receive formal pictures taken at school/clubs and contribute financially to their wellbeing. They are also usually the gateway to their extended family and support the children to have relationships with grandparents, etc. In addition, they attempt to be available in a supporting role and can attend medical appointments, etc.

When PA is involved, over time, the non-resident parent often becomes the 'targeted parent', and a hostile situation begins, whereby the alienating parent starts to interfere with the child's relationship with the targeted parent. In my experience, the eldest child resists contact with a targeted, non-resident parent before the others, then the second child, etc., until no child attends. Typically, over time the targeted parent realises that the other parent is alienating them from their child, and they may reach out to legal services for support. It is often the case that by the time the targeted parent seeks legal advice, their situation has been deteriorating for many years. They have typically attempted to try to appease the alienating parent, or they have argued with the alienating parent, believing they have recourse to legal support if required.

Research findings suggest that intense marital friction, followed by a difficult separation, in the context of particular features of the child and parents, predicts PA (3). The alienating parent believes the child does not need the targeted parent, and they in turn believe that no one can really help them. In my experience of parents involved in severe parental alienation, the alienating parent usually indicates that they feel the targeted parent relationship is unnecessary for the child and usually they say it is the child who does not want the relationship. Often, they say they have attempted to encourage the child to attend contact; however, the child 'does not want to go'. This is a typical response. The alienating parent usually says, 'if everyone leaves us alone, then we can look at it again in the future'. It is sadly the case that usually 'the future' never arrives and that if the family are left alone as requested, then the relationship with the targeted parent is over. Any emotional distress exhibited by the child is deemed to be caused by the targeted parent's behaviour, words and/or absence/presence. The targeted parent is sometimes surprised by the child's behaviour, and even when the court professionals explain the situation, saying the child does not want to see them, the targeted parent is often confused and in disbelief, particularly if there was a strong positive relationship beforehand.

Discussing whether the targeted parent has contributed to their situation feels a bit like 'victim blaming'; however, there are occasions when a targeted parent has behaved aggressively or poorly, particularly if they are volatile or become overly frustrated with the alienating parent. This of course gives the alienating parent more credibility with professionals and gives them an excuse to phone the police to report the targeted parent's 'aggression' or 'threatening behaviour'. There are occasions when the targeted parent behaves poorly and minimises or dismisses this, expecting the child to forgive them simply because they are a parent. These are not typical of PA cases and could lead to justifiable estrangement, which is discussed in Chapter 4.

Staying with the 'victim blaming' theme, it has been reported that targeted parents may contribute to their situation by being passive, rejecting the child, being immature or self-focused, placing unreasonable demands on the child or displaying little empathy towards them; however, this has not usually been my experience with these cases, and the presentation may have changed during the 20 years since research to show this was produced (4). Attempts to identify the causes of PA have found that often there is a 'hybrid' situation, whereby a child is exposed to denigration of the targeted parent in the context of some real limitations in parenting by the targeted parent (5). There are occasions when the targeted parent presents as overly confident about their relationship with the child and/or their parenting skills. This sometimes happens because the targeted parent no longer lives with the child and is not aware of changes that are taking place as the child matures, and so they try to manage the child they knew before contact broke down. Typically, by the time the targeted parent sees the child again, which sometimes takes years, the child has matured and changed, so the targeted parent has to get to know them again. The targeted parent does not always think this through and so they present as clumsy and uninformed about their child. There are also occasions when a targeted parent is psychologically minded and has thought about their child's development without professional intervention. They are prepared and intent on not making a mistake. They consider the child's experiences and are excited about getting to know their child again.

Problems with the literature

Although there have been significant efforts to try to consider the emotional impact of PA on targeted parents, many of the studies have had small sample sizes enabling only qualitative data, or the parents have self-identified as targeted parents (6–7). The lack of data reflects the difficulty with recruitment and permissions for researchers attempting to describe this group, rather than a lack of interest in the subject area.

Gender differences

It appears that only two studies have looked at targeted mothers specifically (8–9). The first study had one mother, and the second had nine (8–9). The second study, conducted in Israel, considered the experience of motherhood for self-identified alienated mothers and found that they felt they had been exploited by their partners, who were male in this study, and the fathers used the children to hurt them (9). It was concluded that the mothers in this study were traumatised by their experiences, and being told they were 'bad mothers' exacerbated their own fears about their parenting ability. As a result of their experiences, they did not recover and adjust; rather, they felt deprived and alone. Most of the women in this Israeli study used marriage as a vehicle from which to leave their home, and it is not clear whether this reflected a dependency on the males; however, it is an example of how individuals can be harmed by PA.

It is likely that one of the reasons for the small number of studies is because historically most children remained with their mother after parental separation, and a lot of PA writing was based on the premise that the mother was the resident parent (referred to as the 'custodial' parent in the US) and the father the non-resident parent, who, in an ideal world, had regular contact with their child (different rules are likely to have applied for same-gender or gender non-specific parents). The situation required both parents to be prepared to put their differences aside for the benefit of their child and work together. Whilst it remains the case today that mothers more usually become the resident parent after separation, there is an increase in single male/female parents, same-gender parents or co-parents with new partners in blended families, and this change in society has to be considered a factor when looking at these cases.

There are findings of improved life satisfaction scores when joint residential arrangements are successful, with both parents reporting more leisure time, mothers enjoying more employment opportunities and romantic relationships, and fathers having better relationships with their children than non-resident fathers (10). Although these findings demonstrate the benefits of successful joint residential arrangements, many parents find themselves in situations where they are unable to do this.

In an online survey of 225 self-identified targeted parents, it was found that targeted mothers are exposed to much higher levels of PA than targeted fathers, with targeted parents feeling threatened by the alienating parent (6). Alienating fathers presented as more aggressive when attempting to reduce the target mother's influence on their children. Tactics included interrogating the child, speaking negatively about the targeted parent, withdrawal of love from the child if they expressed positive feelings about the targeted parent, demanding that the child should be loyal to them, developing an alliance with the child that was considered unhealthy, disclosing negative information about the targeted parent and encouraging the child to be difficult when with the targeted parent. Another study (11) where 72 couples were examined, i.e. 144 participants, had similar findings, and the researchers identified that in 90% of alienation cases, targeted parents did not receive information about the child; disrespectful behaviours towards the targeted parent were rewarded by the alienating parent; and the alienating parent made decisions without consulting the targeted parent, belittled them and prevented them from visiting the children. In 80% – 90% of cases, the following strategies were used:

- Intense questioning after contact.
- Sharing information about the court process.
- Interfering in the child's contact with the targeted parent.
- Hindering telephone contact.
- Using other caregivers without consulting the targeted parent.
- Seeking accomplices, i.e. a new partner or an extended family.

Other strategies, such as changing the child's address without consulting the targeted parent or trying to change the child's surname, were found in less than 20% of cases of PA. In a study of college students and their parents, it was found that students remembered both parents denigrating each other, although divorced parents tended to describe themselves as less denigrating than the children remembered (12). It was felt that parents may have difficulty identifying their own negative behaviours and that children may be better able to report parental denigration (12).

There are also findings that the children involved were more likely to present as challenging when the alienating parent was a father and that mothers were more likely to speak negatively about the father in the presence of the child (11). This is consistent with my clinical experience, where alienating fathers have tended to present as more assertive and vocal about their views and less willing to reflect on the mother's role in their child's life, mostly presenting as dismissive of this or minimising it.

Research has found no difference between genders in the level of alienation described (13), although there was an expectation that mothers would present with more alienating behaviours than fathers (14). More recently, there have been findings that mothers are more likely to use indirect PA behaviours, whereas fathers use both direct and indirect methods (15), although interestingly, fathers' use of direct methods was similar to that of mothers (15).

It has been concluded that the role of gender is unclear, and in the past, mothers may have been more likely to present as alienating parents, but over time, as parenting roles have become less defined, either gender parent can present as the alienator or targeted parent (16). This is consistent with my experience, and I feel that as gender roles continue to become less assigned in some parts of society, the argument about alienating parents being mothers will dissipate.

Emotional impact on the targeted parent

It has been reported that targeted parents are vulnerable to anxiety and depression and tend to be passive (17). They were found to try to avoid conflict with the alienating parent, who held all the power. Other studies found feelings of anger and frustration were prevalent, as was powerlessness, which makes sense (18). In a review of the available literature about targeted parents, it was reported that they felt like victims and that their relationships with their children had been undermined, leading to feelings of isolation, hopelessness and frustration (16).

In another study that spoke to only six fathers, there were findings that targeted parents reported having experienced a traumatic incident when their children were removed from their lives (19). Another study found that targeted parents felt that they had experienced an injustice (3). They expressed concern about not being able to participate in the child's traditions, for example, birthdays, school celebrations, etc. They also felt that formal services were not in place to support them, and they were alone with their discomfort. These descriptions from targeted parents are consistent with each other and with the experiences of many who are subjected to PA.

Impact of the breakdown

Research findings indicate that unsurprisingly, many separated parents experience elevated mental health scores and require intervention (20–21). Taken at face value, we might assume that parental separation leads to impairment in mental health, and it seems entirely possible, if not likely, that parents who experience relationship breakdown will suffer emotionally; however, it is also possible that people who have mental health and/or personality problems have poor relationships with others, and this leads to a greater incidence of separation. Whilst mental illness and relationships are bidirectional, i.e. they have an impact on each other, there are findings that a good relationship can have a positive effect on mental health, whereas the influence of an individual's emotional welfare on their relationships is weaker (22). Being a parent is likely to place additional stresses and strains on an already fragile relationship, and a separated parent has a lot to try to contend with, in terms of making arrangements to see their children and trying to negotiate a precarious situation with an often equally or more unhappy ex-partner.

Following findings of significant levels of mental illness in the parents of children attending services for support with mental health issues (23), there has been considerable effort put into how to intervene to help parents and how this can have a positive effect on the mental health of their children (24–25). One study found that 33–36% of parents of children with mental health problems had significant issues themselves, and treatment of these issues had a positive impact on the child involved. This study highlighted the importance of treating the child in the context of their family environment (24).

In relation to families, it is not only parents going through a difficult relationship break-up who are likely to experience emotional disturbance whilst they adjust to their change in circumstances. It is the same for their children, who have to accept a different family set-up, whilst they also usually have to go along with their parents' decision-making about who they will live with and what contact arrangements will be in place. There have been reports that parents sometimes work to align their children with themselves at this time, resulting in the child having problems with the non-resident parent after separation and leading to PA.

Parents who do not have contact

Parents who do not have contact with their children after separation have been reported to experience higher rates depression than their peers, and it is the quality of the parent-child relationship that impacts on parental mental health, with fathers expressing more distress if they have conflict with the mother, do not speak to their child or feel they have lost their father role (26). Most people experience high levels of stress when they are going through a relationship breakdown, and this is normal; however, when children are involved, this makes the experience even more complex and challenging.

In Sweden, it is reported that 10% of school-age children live between both parents (27), and it is considered that 35% of children whose parents do not live together reside with both parents. In a large study of 9225 parents, there were findings that families with two biological parents living together were significantly less likely to experience mental health problems than either of the parents if they were single. When mothers met a new partner, they remained significantly more likely to experience anxiety and worry than fathers. Interestingly, there are findings that joint residence is associated with more mental health problems for mothers (28), which seems like a significant finding for gender issues and PA research. It was suggested that this may result from parents missing the child, particularly if mothers assume the bulk of the parenting when they are in a two-parent biological family (this study assumed that each family had a mother and a father) (28). For single parents, it was considered possible that the stress associated with moving children from one home to another and constantly adjusting to their situation was likely to be difficult and ultimately impact on mental health. The authors recognised that they did not control for the period of time since separation, and parents may recover over time once they have gone through an adjustment period. It also seemed that the researchers did not control for pre-child mental health problems, i.e. the parents may have been vulnerable and experienced mental health problems not associated with parenting at all. In addition, this research seems contrary to the findings about life satisfaction, although that may have related to successful joint residence situations as opposed to those involving conflict/and or stress (28).

Targeted parents experience high levels of stress associated with their situation, and alienation can have a negative effect on their mental health, with increased incidence of anxiety and depression reported (6). At times, stress is exhibited by physical health issues, including fatigue and weight loss (3, 7, 29). Also, targeted parents have reported feelings of despair and dissatisfaction with the support services available to them (16). There is often a lack of formal support for parents who have been alienated from their children. If they are accused of aggression or worse, they are left feeling persecuted and alone, and it is usually only family and friends who really know them who offer the support they need (3). Despite that, they often employ appropriate coping strategies. Targeted parents have to try to cope with wondering if they could do anything to stop or prevent the alienating parent from denigrating them or making the situation worse, whilst at the same time think about improving their relationship with their child. It is therefore particularly difficult to try to adjust to their situation when the difficulties persist.

It was found that targeted parents employed a range of techniques to support resilience, including both individual and community practices, and the resarchers' findings support the notion that resilience teaching is likely to be an area of consideration for intervention (30). Studies showed that targeted parents tended to be emotionally resilient and used appropriate coping strategies, such as education, social support and being stoic, and one qualitative study found parents expressed feelings of unconditional love towards their children, which helped them cope with their situation (3, 7). They categorised targeted parents' coping strategies into two forms: emotion-focused, for example finding distractions, seeking therapeutic services and inhibiting emotional responses to alienating behaviours; and problem-focused, for example trying to get close to the child through their network, information seeking or indirect contact (3, 7).

In my experience targeted parents want to present as fit, emotionally healthy and able to parent. They attempt to be seen as stable in the event that the alienating parent may use any vulnerability as a 'reason' to reduce or stop contact. In addition to assessing mental health using a standardised measure, professionals who are appropriately qualified could review the medical records to ensure that no underlying mental health condition exists likely to impact on parenting. There are also occasions when targeted parents feel so poorly that they require psychopharmacological intervention, and below is an excerpt from the GP notes and records of a targeted parent (with permission to share):

> was at Social Services meeting yesterday. . . . Is going back to Court about custody of his children. A lot of pressure. He cannot take it anymore. Feels lies are being told. No one is listening to him. Was very stressed by it. Pain in

chest and into neck – put it down to tension and stress. Hasn't been sleeping well. Head feels scrambled. Went to work today but had to leave. Feels overwhelmed by it all. Has seen children for around 2 hours in the last 2 years. He says this is all [his ex's] doing. He says that [his ex] reports that the kids feel he has walked out on them, when this is not the case . . . agreed [to antidepressant medication and is] aware of risk of worsening anxiety in short term and of possibility of suicidal ideation.

One publication reported that targeted parents experienced great suffering (which is consistent with my experiences) and that when they are asked to leave the situation alone, sometimes they did so and never saw the child again (31). It was noted that sometimes when parents attended for intervention, they reported feeling regret that they had not acted sooner and helpless for trying to approach the issue much later (31).

A question that arises is whether targeted parents should have contact with their children, if they have behaved violently towards the alienating parent. There are consistent findings that if children are exposed to violence, they are more likely to have emotional and behavioural disturbance (32), and ultimately, the child's safety is more important than meeting their need for contact with their absent parent; however, this is a separate and complex area, and much depends on whether the parent has been assessed as presenting a risk to the child.

Personality

One possible consideration for PA research is whether there is a particular personality type that's more likely to be targeted than others. In a study of six targeted parents, five fathers and one mother, only a weak association was found relating to personality characteristics and potential for PA (8), but another study found that targeted parents had a milder pattern of conformity and conventionality and were more flexible in their thinking than other parents (1). The targeted parents described themselves as adjusted and were able to manage their situation.

A review of nine studies on targeted parents found that they did not tend to present with disturbance in personality (16). Overall, targeted parents tended to consider themselves competent parents and effective disciplinarians, felt they set healthy boundaries whilst encouraging independence, and held a positive attitude towards their role (16).

In my experience there are also targeted parents who give up and walk away. They mostly cite the impact of the conflict on the child, although if they have second families, they then have to consider how many resources they can attribute to their situation when they are needed by their new family. Another comment I have heard from targeted parents is that they cannot justify the cost of legal involvement, and this seems to be particularly the case when they have a second family.

Grandparents and extended family

Usually when the relationship between the targeted, non-resident parent and the children deteriorates, then contact with the non-resident extended family is lost too, and in a study of 173 children, it was found that 20 years after parental separation, the relationships with these family groups were poor or non-existent (33). Also, in separated families where the mother was the resident parent, there have been findings that children were more likely to be close to the paternal grandmother only if the mother maintained her own relationship with the paternal grandmother (34). Therefore, if a parent is targeted, then so, too, is the extended family of aunts, uncles, cousins and grandparents, although this varies. Sometimes, if the targeted parent does not have an amicable relationship with a particular family member, then they become aligned with an alienating parent, even helping them by writing negative letters to the court about the targeted parent or providing information to professionals that reflects their history of grievance with the targeted parent. In my experience, it is not usual for a targeted parent who has a positive relationship with a family member to find that the family member has a good relationship with the alienating parent, and both families often 'take sides' in any conflict. Targeted grandparents often find alienation particularly difficult to cope with, especially if they were close to the child before the parents separated. Targeted grandparents are often devastated if they have been very involved with the children before the parental separation and suddenly find they are no longer part of their lives and do not attend school productions, religious events, etc. Quite often when I see children, the extended family are demonised and have become part of the child's perception of what constitutes the problem.

Conclusion

The targeted parent can be considered totally, partially or not remotely responsible for their situation. If the targeted parent is partially responsible for their situation, then this is referred to as a 'hybrid' situation. When there is some contribution by the targeted parent, it may involve them exposing their children to language and/ or behaviour that causes their child discomfort and makes the alienating parent's task that much easier. Sometimes it is the case that the child observed conflict in the home during the parental separation, and this led them to feel more aligned with the alienating parent, with the targeted parent struggling to understand why their child is upset with them.

References

1   Roma, P., Marchetti, D., Mazza, C., Burla, F. and Verrocchio, M.C. (2020). MMPI profiles of mothers engaged in parental alienation. *Journal of Family Issues*. doi:10.1177/ 0192513X20918393.

2 Warshak, R.A. (2013). Severe cases of parental alienation. In D. Lorandos, W. Bernet and S.R. Sauber (Eds.), *American series in behavioral science and law. Parental alienation: The handbook for mental health and legal professionals* (pp. 125–162). Springfield, IL: Charles C. Thomas Publisher.

3 Tavares, A., Crespo, C. and Ribeiro, M.T. (2021). What does it mean to be a target parent? Parents' experiences in the context of parental alienation. *Journal of Child and Family Studies*. doi:10.1007/s10826-021-01914-6.

4 Kelly, J.B. and Johnston, J.R. (2001). The alienated child: A reformulation of parental alienation syndrome. *Family Court Review*, 39, 249–266. doi:10/1111/k.174-1617.2001. tb00609.x.

5 Garber, B.A. (2011). Parental alienation and the dynamics of the enmeshed parent-child dyad: Adultification, parentification and infantilization. *Family Court Review*, 49, 322–335.

6 Balmer, S., Matthewson, M. and Haines, J. (2018). Parental alienation: Targeted parent perspective. *Australian Journal of Psychology*. doi:10.1111/ajpy.12159.

7 Poustie, C., Matthewson, M. and Balmer, S. (2018). The forgotten parent: The targeted parent perspective of parental alienation. *Journal of Family Issues*. doi:10.1177/0192513X187778867.

8 Vassiliou, D. and Cartwright, G.F. (2001). The lost parents' perspective on parental alienation syndrome. *American Journal of Family Therapy*, 29, 181–191. doi:10.1080/019261801750424307.

9 Finzi-Dottan, R., Goldblatt, H. and Cohen-Masica, O. (2012). The experience of motherhood for alienated mothers. *Child and Family Social Work*, 17, 316–325. doi:10.1111/j.1365-2206.2011.00782.x.

10 Van der Heijden, F., Gähler, M. and Härkönen, J. (2015). Are parents with shared residence happier? Children's post-divorce residence arrangements and parents' life satisfaction. *Stockholm Research Reports in Demography*, 2015, 17.

11 López, T.J., Iglesias, V.E.N. and García, P.F. (2014). Parental alienation gradient: Strategies for a syndrome. *The American Journal of Family Therapy*, 42. doi:10.1080/01926187.2013.820116.

12 Rowen, J. and Emery, R.E. (2019). Parental denigration reports across parent-child dyads: Divorced parents underreport denigration behaviours compared to children. *Journal of Child Custody*, 16, 197–208.

13 Harman, J.J., Leder-Elder, S. and Biringen, Z. (2016). Prevalence of parental alienation drawn from a representative poll. *Children and Youth Services Review*, 66, 62–66.

14 Harman, J.J., Biringen, Z., Ratajack, E.M., Outland, P.L. and Kraus, A. (2016). Parents behaving badly: Gender biases in the perception of parental alienating behaviors. *Journal of Family Psychology*, 30, 866–874. doi:10.1037/Fam0000232.

15 Harman, J.J., Lorandos, D., Biringen, Z. and Grubb, C. (2020). Gender differences in the use of parental alienating behaviors. *Journal of Family Violence*, 35, 459–469. doi:10.1007/s10896-019-00097-5.

16 Maturana, S.L., Matthewson, M., Dwan, C. and Norris, K. (2018). Characteristics and experiences of targeted parents of parental alienation from their own perspective: A systematic literature review. *Australian Journal of Psychology*. doi:10.1111/ajpy.12226.

17 Kopetski, L. (1998). Identifying cases of parental alienation syndrome – part II. *The Colorado Lawyer*, 27, 61–64.

18   Baker, A.J.L. (2010). Even when you win you lose: Targeted parents' perception of their attorneys. *The American Journal of Family Therapy*, 38, 292–309.

19   Bosch-Brits, M., Wessels, C. and Roux, A. (2018). Fathers' experience and perceptions of parental alienation in high-conflict divorce. *Social Work*, 54. doi:10.15270/54-1-617.

20   Keating, A., Sharry, J., Murphy, M., Rooney, B. and Carr, A. (2015). An evaluation of the Parents Plus – Parenting when Separated programme. *Clinical Child Psychology and Psychiatry*. doi:10.1177/1359104515581717.

21   Novo, M., Fariña, F., Seijo, D., Vázquez, M.J. and Arce, R. (2019). Assessing the effects of an education program on mental health problems in separated parents. *Psicothema*, 31, 284–291. doi:10.7334/psicothema2018.299.

22   Braithwaite, S. and Holt-Lunstad, J. (2017). Romantic relationships and mental health. *Current Opinion in Psychology*, 13, 120–125. doi:10.1016/j.copsych.2016.04.001.

23   Wesseldijk, L.W., Dielemann, G.C., van Steensel, F.J.A., Bartels, M., Hudziak, J.J., Lindauer, R.J.L., Bögels, S.M. and Middeldorp, C.M. (2018). Risk factors for parental psychopathology: A study in families with children or adolescents with psychopathology. *European Child and Adolescent Psychiatry*, 27, 1575–1584. doi:10.1007/s00787-018-1156-6.

24   Campbell, T.C.H., Reupert, R.A., Sutton, K., Basu, S., Davidson, G., Middeldorp, C.M., Naughton, M. and Maybery, D. (2020). Prevalence of mental illness among parents of children receiving treatment within child and adolescent mental health services (CAMHS): A scoping review. *European Child and Adolescent Psychiatry*. doi:10.1007/s00787-020-01502-x.

25   Reupert, A., Price-Robertson, R. and Maybery, D. (2021). Parenting as a focus of recovery: A systematic review of current practice. *Psychiatric Rehabilitation Journal*, 40, 361–370. doi:10.1037/prj0000240.

26   Vogt Yuan, A.S. (2014). Father-child relationship and non-resident fathers' psychological distress: What helps and what hurts? *Journal of Family Issues*. doi:10.1177/0192513X14526394.

27   Bergström, M., Modin, B., Fransson, E., Rajmil, L., Berlin, M., Gustafsson, P.A. and Hjern, A. (2013). Living in two homes – a Swedish national survey of wellbeing in 12- and 15-year-olds with joint physical custody. *BMC Public Health*, 13, 868. doi:10.1186/1471-2458-13-868.

28   Fritzell, S., Gähler, M. and Fransson, E. (2020). Child living arrangements following separation and mental health of parents in Sweden. *Social Science and Medicine (SSM) Population Health*, 10. doi:10.1016/j.ssmph.2019.100511.

29   Torun, F., Torun, S.D. and Matthewson, M. (2021). Parental alienation: Targeted parent experience in Turkey. *The American Journal of Family Therapy*. doi:10.1080/0192 6187.2021.1895903.

30   Scharp, K.M., Kubler, K.F. and Wang, T.R. (2020). Individual and community practices for constructing communicative resilience: Exploring the communicative processes or coping with parental alienation. *Journal of Applied Communication Research*, 48, 207–226. doi:10/1080/00909882.2020.1734225.

31   Lowenstein, L.F. (2015). What can yet be done with older children who have been long-term victims of parental alienation? *Journal of Divorce and Remarriage*, 56, 513–515. doi:10.1080/10502556.2015.1060822.

32 Holt, S., Buckley, H. and Whelan, S. (2008). The impact of exposure to domestic violence on children and young people: A review of the literature. *Child Abuse and Neglect*, 8, 797–810. doi:10.1016/j.chiabu.2008.02.004.

33 Ahrons, C.R. (2007). Family ties after divorce: Long-term implications for children. *Family Process*, 46, 53–65. doi:10.1111/j.1545–5300.2006.00191.x.

34 Attar-Schwartz, S. and Fuller-Thomson, E. (2017). Adolescents' closeness to paternal grandmothers in the face of parents' divorce. *Children and Youth Services Review*, 77, 118–126. doi:10.1016/j.childyouth.2017.04.008.

Chapter 7

The alienated child

Introduction

Parental separation can have a negative effect on all aspects of a child's function-ing, and although differences between children have been observed, there have been findings of increased mental health and emotional problems, behavioural disorders, reduced social skills and impairment in academic attainment (1–5). It is likely the outcome depends on the child's experiences and level of resilience. In addition, there are findings that children who experience parental separation grow up with an increased likelihood of functioning more poorly as parents them-selves (6). In research relating to maintaining relationships, it was found that chil-dren who maintained relationships with their non-resident parent (the father in this study) tended to have better relationships with both their absent parent and the resident parent and enjoyed a more productive social life than children who did not have contact with their non-resident parent (7). In another study it was noted that the more involved fathers were with their child prior to family separation, the more likely they were to remain in contact afterwards (8). This study found that as time went on it became increasingly difficult for fathers to maintain relationships with their children with the same intensity, which makes sense if they do not have the same level of contact as the resident parent. Research on 303 high-conflict separated parents who volunteered for the study found that parental emotional sta-bility, good mental health and good shared parenting arrangements were linked to a more positive outcome for children and resulted in fewer emotional difficulties in children involved in cases where a high level of symptomatology was exhibited in parents with little sharing of the parenting role (9).

It is therefore generally agreed that the best outcome for children following parental separation is for amicable co-parenting and shared care arrangements, and there is substantial research to support this (for a review see (10)). The child spends as much time with one parent as they do with another, and if one or both parents work, then they put supports in place to help the child and ensure their need to have a relationship with both parents is met. Amicable co-parenting has been found to have a positive effect on child functioning, and when an improve-ment in co-parenting has been achieved, better child adjustment is observed (11).

DOI: 10.4324/9781003156147-7

However, shared care arrangements are not without their challenges for families, both for the parents and for the children. Some young children have described feeling overwhelmed when they come out of school to different family members, not knowing which home they are going to on any particular day, whilst others are completely comfortable with being collected by a range of people if that is the situation; some children even enjoy it. A lot depends on the child and their relationships with the individuals who are collecting them. Likewise, parents may have to negotiate with each other for pick-ups and drop-offs on different days, which can be difficult at times, although a good shared-care arrangement can have significant advantages for parents, too, particularly when there is good support and flexibility around afterschool and weekend/holiday childcare routines.

Although they are not directly comparable, in considering whether it is the actual parental absence from the home that impacts on children, studies show that 'left-behind' children of parents who migrated, usually for economic purposes (one in seven individuals in the world is a migrant, and the number is increasing globally), have been found to have an 85% increased risk of anxiety, 52% increased risk of depression, 70% increased risk of suicidal ideation, 24% increased risk of substance misuse and also some physical health issues when both parents migrated (12). This was a review of 111 studies, which altogether reflected on the impact of parental migration on 264,967 children, and it was concluded that parental migration is detrimental to children. This study indicates the significant impact separating a child from their parent can have.

Parents who are physically present but lack capacity to engage with parenting due to emotional disturbance have also been the subject of research. It is widely recognised that children's needs are best met by parents who are emotionally stable and that parents with mental health problems are more likely to have children with psychiatric and neurodevelopmental issues (13–14).

A parent can be absent from the home because of work/military service or incarceration, and there is increased recognition that these situations must be addressed appropriately to prevent a negative impact on any child involved (15–16). Other reasons for parental absence relate to illness or death, and the research examining the impact on a child when one parent dies shows an increased risk of mental health challenges as well as other impairment in functioning (17–18). Investigators noted that there are many factors to consider, e.g. the resilience and age of the child, the level of care they are receiving and whether they have to move house, school, etc. This suggests that it is the overall impact on the child, in the context of their having to manage social issues, etc., that needs to be considered. In this context, there may be other issues associated with the remaining parent's ability to also adjust to loss and their capacity to parent their child during a period of grief.

Pre- and post-separation experiences are likely to impact on the child, and it is usually the case that the more adverse events encountered, the more difficult it is for children to grow up without experiencing emotional disturbance. Having at least one stable parent is helpful, and although it does not always happen, it is better for the child if the more empathic and caring parent is the resident parent after separation. If this is the case, it is likely they will have contact with their non-resident parent. In the case of alienation, the more entrenched the alienating parent is and the less contact the child is given, the more harm is likely to result. Interestingly, there have been findings that even when the contact was of poor quality after parental separation (the study was with fathers), this still had a better impact on children's life satisfaction and health than no contact at all. In this significant study of 4207 children, it was found that 40% had poor communication with their father after separation, and 10% had no contact at all (19).

The process of alienation from the child's viewpoint

Considerable effort has gone into thinking about how a child can become so strongly aligned with an alienating parent, and it has been reported that because the alienating parent is typically the primary carer, the child trusts the perceptions of the alienating parent more than they trust their own (20). They do not have the relationship with the targeted parent to correct any misperceptions. The child is then terrified of leaving the one 'safe' person that they know exists. One study found that alienated children perceived that the alienating parent's emotional survival or their relationship with the alienating parent was dependent on them rejecting the targeted parent (21). Another study noted that the alienating parent applied pressure to the child so that they felt they had to develop an alliance with them (22). It has been reported that it is relatively easy to alienate a child, since they can easily blur facts and feelings, and alienating parents exploit the emotion, for example, if a targeted parent feels they have to say 'no' to a child or discipline them in some way, then when they return to the care of the alienating parent, they can be reminded of any negative experiences with the targeted parent. Alienating parents can then exaggerate how difficult it felt for the child to have the targeted parent say 'no' to them (20).

Research into the impact of one parent denigrating the other has shown that young adults sometimes dislike the behaviour of the denigrating parent as much as, or more than, the one being denigrated (22). This seems to cast doubt on the idea of a parent alienating a child partly through denigration. In this study it was not clear whether the young people involved had relationships with their denigrated parent before their parents separated, and it seemed the study reflected the relationship with the resident parent rather than alienation issues. It would be interesting to assess school-aged children involved in situations where PA had been raised as an issue, using the same denigration measures to see whether these results still applied. Notably, young adults with a denigrating parent were more likely to experience depression and have poorer life satisfaction, which reflects the negative impact of parental denigration on a child.

Also relevant to the denigration research, there are findings that children were more apprehensive during communication with caregivers in adulthood if they had experienced PA in childhood, so the experience had a significant impact on their functioning (23). Similarly, researchers carried out a study that administered a questionnaire to 205 college students to assess exposure to alienating communication from their caregivers when they were approximately eight to 12 years old (24). They found negative comments about the other parent impacted on the child's relationship with the denigrating parent *as well as* with the targeted parent. Those with better self-esteem were more likely to have a relationship with the targeted parent when they became adults. This study found no relationship between current self-esteem, depression and memories of PA from childhood (24).

Fears and phobias

Social learning theory describes how an individual learns a fear response, and it has been reported that emotions have three response systems: physiological states, behavioural changes, and more subjective responses and cognitions associated with the states, i.e. verbal-cognitive responses (25–26). It is usual for children to have some fears, and a literature review has found that most children aged between four and 19 years old average between two and five fears (27), although one study found an average of 14 fears per child (28). These fears tend to be fairly benign and typically involve the dark, spiders, snakes, etc. Genetics contributes to the development of fears, and a child can be predisposed to experience this phenomenon, or they are taught fears in their environment, known as vicarious fears. There are findings that a substantial proportion of fear is related to stimuli present in the environment (29).

Vicarious fear can also be learned by observing another person's fearful reaction to a stimulus or situation, for example observing screaming when a person saw a spider. This could be the process by which fear is learned in PA (30). There are encouraging studies to show that fear can also be unlearned in the same manner, which could be an area for rehabilitation if the alienating parent was agreeable (31). Fear can also be learned by what we hear or see, and studies have shown that parents frequently share information about threatening stimuli or situations and that this can induce fear in children (32). Therefore, if the alienating parent is genuinely frightened of the targeted parent, this can induce fear in the child without recognition from the adult that this is happening. There are indications that some children might be more receptive than others to observational or vicarious learning (33). These considerations emphasise the necessity for an individual approach to cases.

Memory and suggestibility

A child may be prompted to have memories of events that have not actually occurred, and in situations where PA is present, children might describe memories of situations they were unlikely to remember because of their age at the time of the alleged incident; for example, many children say that one of the reasons they do not want to see the targeted parent is because they mistreated them when they were living with them. Often children say they remember negative events, for example things that happened when they were a baby that they could not possibly remember. Some children are quite sure that they remember this event, and others say they overheard other adults in the family refer to it.

The memories of children can be influenced and altered by misinformation, misleading stories and emotional pressure to please an alienating parent. This is particularly the case when children are young, and children do not begin to remember events reliably until they are at least three-and-a-half to four years old (34). Children are more suggestible than adults, and the level of suggestibility reduces as they become older. It is believed this is likely to be associated with improved memory as they mature (35), and this supports the descriptions given by other researchers, who stated that the younger the child was, the easier it was to manipulate them (20).

There is a general consensus that children can have false memories of childhood sexual assault (CSA) and that the impact of this is traumatic (36). When children have experienced CSA, they are more likely to be re-victimised as adults (37–38), and there are other long-term implications for an individual's social, emotional, cognitive and behavioural functioning. Despite this, many alienating parents allege sexual abuse without apparently having knowledge of the implications for their child.

There are findings that children who have experienced sexual assault trauma are more likely to change their opinions when under duress and also that if a family member was involved, then trauma symptoms were more severe, and the child was more vulnerable to giving erroneous information (39). There are also findings that children who have trauma symptoms are more likely to incorporate misleading information into memory if they are exposed to leading questions (40). This highlights the need for appropriate assessment, informed by what is known about child memory and suggestibility.

Problems with the literature on parental alienation

It is recognised that although it is well-established that divorce/parental separation has a negative impact on children, PA may be present yet unidentified (41). This means that research indicating the problems associated with parental separation might to some extent reflect the impact of PA. It is difficult to study alienated children since they do not often engage with professionals, particularly if they are in the care of the alienating parent; then even if PA is agreed on by all the legal teams involved, the family may not agree to participate in research. Most of the studies looking at the long-term implications of PA have been carried out retrospectively on college students or adults who report they were alienated as children. There have been thorough attempts by researchers to identify adults who were alienated as children, although they are reliant on the memory of the participants who report they had this experience. More studies of alienated children are required for evaluators to be confident when they are speaking about the long-term effects of PA, particularly if they are carrying out follow-up studies some years later.

What it is like to be an alienated child

A child can reject a parent for a range of possible reasons, which may not necessarily be associated with PA, and most investigators considering the issues associated with PA are aware of hybrid situations that can be a combination of both the alienating and targeted behaviours that impact on the child. In addition, there might be other reasons, such as the child's personality (42). Although the child and the alienating parent often offer a number of 'reasons' for the child's decision not to have contact with their targeted parent, in many cases of PA the child has not seen the targeted parent for a long time, sometimes years, and so the parent has not had an opportunity to do anything to upset the child. The rejection is, therefore, associated with the child's memory of the targeted parent or the alienating parent maintaining negative thoughts relating to the absent parent.

The alienated child is often angry and typically expresses no empathy for the targeted parent, which raises a concern about the impact of PA on their personality and future relationships. If children are being taught to ignore the distress of their other parent, then they are learning not to have empathy for others. One study reported an adult saying, 'I was a horrible, horrible person' and another saying 'I feel really bad that I did that' to the targeted parent, and individuals have to live with any shame and guilt attached to their behaviour (43). Alternatively, the child may feel no shame or guilt for mistreating another person, and then the professionals have to consider the impact of their behaviours on their personality. It is of course entirely possible that they may have lacked empathy for others anyway, particularly if one of the parents has deficits in this feature of personality. In addition, the child is ignoring their own need to have a relationship with their other parent and also learning that their welfare is not as important as the alienating parent's.

Alienated children might have a difficult relationship with the alienating parent and have been found to be overly dependent, particularly for their age (44). In terms of patterns of behaviours, usually if there is more than one child, the eldest child stops attending contact, then the next eldest, etc., until contact no longer takes place with any of the children.

Some have noted that in cases of PA there is no positive narrative about the absent parent that the child can enjoy, and their birthdays and special days, like Father's or Mother's Day, are not celebrated with them, although they might be enjoyed with a new partner (45). The absent parent is sometimes referred to by their first or another derogatory name by both the alienating parent and their children, who want desperately to align themselves with the alienating parent, and photographs and other signs of the absent parent are not evident in the home of an alienating parent.

Alienated children may not be told about the absent parent's attempts to contact them, and they may have no awareness of attempts at indirect or direct contact, i.e. gifts or cards that are thrown out, phone/video calls not responded to or scheduled contact that is missed. Court attendances may never be mentioned, and so the child believes that the absent parent has not attempted to contact them, or if the child is aware of court attendances, these are communicated as negative events, brought about by the targeted parent to create difficulty for the alienating parent. Children often know much more about court and adult affairs than they would be expected to know or should know, as typically it causes them worry and distress, and children say that they are worried that their alienating parent might go to prison because the targeted parent has taken them to court. The targeted parent is therefore perceived as 'the problem' because they have caused the distress by bringing the case before the court.

The impact of feeling rejected by an absent parent

Alienating parents often profess a strong positive relationship with their own parents, although they resist any attempt to help them understand the likely impact on their child of not having a relationship with the targeted family. The alienated child often believes that the absent or targeted parent did not wish to have a relationship with them. There is significant research that shows poor psychological adjustment in adults who were rejected by parents (46). Other studies show associations between parental rejection and depressed mood, in addition to other significant mental health conditions (47).

Adults often say they had an absent parent who 'never bothered' with them. They usually say this in an angry or disappointed manner and, when asked, say they feel upset that they had a parent who did not care about them. Sometimes they have siblings with different fathers who have all rejected them, and this raises the question about why a number of different parents from one family all decided not to engage with their children. It is entirely possible that one parent had relationships with people who did not want to remain in contact with their children, but it raises an issue about whether all partners involved with the resident parent chose to reject their children. If a parent asks to see a child after a period of no contact, then some consideration has to be given to the reasons for their absence and their understanding about the responsibility associated with coming back into the child's life. The impact on the child is the focus of any thinking about re-establishing relationships after a period of no contact.

Emotional impact of parental alienation

It has been established that children of divorce are mainly impacted on by the relationship between their parents, post-separation parenting and the parent-child relationship quality. There are findings that children of divorced parents had more difficulty adjusting when they were exposed to negative parental behaviours (48). In a meta-analysis (which employs a methodology to consider all the scientific papers relating to a specific question) of 24,854 divorced families, it was found that children involved in high-conflict situations which continued after the divorce or separation were at greater risk of triangulation (involving the child in the argument), parentification (the child becomes parental with the resident parent) and parental disclosure about the relationship (48). It was noted that children of separated parents were more likely to have both internalising and externalising problems, poorer self-esteem and lower social competence than their peers. The study concluded that exposure to conflict and hostility had a negative impact on children, and separately impacted on the parent's capacity to engage with their child, so that they were less attentive and involved than usual. The authors concluded that the quality of post-divorce parenting was important, that negative parenting behaviours after divorce may have a bigger impact on healthy child adjustment than deficiencies in positive parenting and that occasions when the child was involved in the parental dispute or put into an adult role were of concern when hostility continued after the separation, because of the likely poor impact on the child.

Self-esteem in children who share their time between two parents after separation has been found to be higher than for those in lone-parent families, which supports the case for co-parenting (49). Similarly, there are consistent findings of low self-esteem in adults who were exposed to PA when they were children (41, 44, 50). Given that poor self-esteem can impact on an individual's academic and occupational attainment and other important aspects of functioning, there are important implications for young people (51). The child exposed to PA may be told that their other parent did not want them or value them, and this can significantly impact self-esteem (52). The child's connection to the targeted family and their extended family can lead the child to believe that they too are implicated in the alienated parent's negative assertions. Some adults who said they had experienced PA as children later said they felt the 'bad parent' was part of them, and so they struggled with thoughts around this and felt that they must also be 'bad' (43). This was particularly the case for children who bore a physical likeness to their targeted parent, and even more so if they were the same gender. It was noted that negative feelings about themselves were incorporated into their self-worth and had significant implications for their functioning (43).

In a study of six adults who reported they had been alienated from a parent, it was found that prior to the parental separation, the child felt distant from the targeted parent (53). The alienating parent denigrated the targeted parent and 'protected' the children from them. It was noted that as children they felt 'deeply guilty and sad after rejecting the parent', and that as they matured identity was an issue for them (53). The study suggested that even a tenuous link with the targeted parent could sometimes lead to a resolution at a later stage and a re-kindling of the relationship.

Self-esteem in PA has been considered by many researchers, usually in addition to other issues. For example, there are findings that adults who believed they had been exposed to PA were more likely to have problems with attachments, low self-esteem, depression and a lack of trust in others (43, 50, 54). One study found

70% of adults who had been exposed to PA as children had depression, and there was a high prevalence of drug/alcohol issues. In addition, 70% said they had been depressed and/or divorced and were involved in PA with their own children (43). It was noted that it was difficult to separate the impact of parental mental health and divorce from the experience of alienation (54).

It has been suggested that working with children to help them resist the influence of the alienating parent might be helpful (50). Notably, these studies included a control group of people whose parents had divorced, although they maintained a relationship with the non-resident parent and did not feel they were exposed to PA.

Many of the issues raised are also problems for children involved in separated families where PA is not assessed. For example, the issue of poor self-esteem is significant in children of separated families and those involving PA, and there are findings that problematic internet use (PIU), i.e. watching inappropriate content or spending too much time on the internet, is more prevalent when adolescents are in separated families and have low self-esteem (55). It makes sense that children who are trying to escape difficult family situations are more likely to get involved in PIU, which increases the likelihood of this becoming an issue in PA.

Social relationships

Attachment relationships provide a 'secure base' from which to engage with others around us. They begin after birth and provide a model which we apply to future relationships. Those who feel safe and secure in their attachment relationships can explore the world and are able to engage with others in a healthy way. Inconsistent, harsh or emotionally inappropriate relationships can result in insecure attachments, which increases the likelihood of poor interpersonal relationships (56). Consistent with the findings of others, it has been found that alienated children were more likely to have insecure attachments and reported that this made them more vulnerable to relationship difficulties (50).

It is noted that a lack of trust is a main issue for alienated children due to trying to believe an alienating parent, who is likely to be indicating to the child that their targeted parent should be rejected without a real reason (57), although the alienating parent might present a reason that is close to the truth. In addition, if the child has previously had a loving relationship with the targeted parent, they may feel their own feelings are untrustworthy. The child might also struggle with thoughts around the alienating parent's narrative if they find it contradicts what they know to be truth, and this teaches them that they cannot trust others, even those closest to them (54).

The 'Alienated Family Relationship Scale' was piloted to consider the perspective of 493 young adults who were involved in conflicted family relationships (58). Seventy-six of the participants were from divorced families, and the other 417 were from intact families. The intention was to consider the impact of one parent's open hostility towards another. Parental conflict was recorded, as well as reports of any alienating exchanges from the parents to each other and similar aspects of the child/parent relationship. It was found that the more frequently young adults perceived alienated relationships within their family, the more distressed and angry they felt towards their parents (58). Results indicated these adults had impairment with both attachments and social relationships. Other studies have reported similar findings (54).

Impact on behaviour

In a study of 38 adults who felt they had been alienated from one parent when they were children, it was found that around one-third had serious difficulty with drugs/and or alcohol (43). Compared with findings that 9.1% of adults in the US have resolved an alcohol/drug problem (59), this suggests the prevalence of alcohol/drug use among adults exposed to PA as children is significantly higher than usual and presents as a particular problem for this group (43).

Cognition

Children with separated parents typically have poorer academic attainment than their peer group, with findings that the older the child was at the time of separation, the greater the magnitude of the damage (3). There is also an association between children's mental health and their academic attainment (60–61), and in addition, poor self-esteem has been found to have a negative impact on academic achievement (62). The implications are that if PA impacts on a child's self-esteem or mental health in the context of their trying to manage any emotional response to a parental separation or conflict over contact, then they are unlikely to perform as well as others in their peer group.

Consistent with this, it was found that PA had a negative impact on educational and occupational attainment, and adult children affected by PA were less likely to complete their education or gain employment by comparison with their peer group (50). It is therefore important to try to reduce the impact of parental separation for children and try to make the transition to single household as seamless as possible.

What harm takes place?

The level of harm is associated with the extent of the alienation. If a child is mildly alienated, there may be very little harm, particularly if the issue does not extend beyond a relatively short period of time. If we assume that a 'severely' alienated child has no contact with the targeted parent and that they are involved in conflict for a number of years, then the harm can include

- Feeling that the targeted parent presents as a threat to them.
- Feeling that by loving the targeted parent they are being disloyal to the alienating parent.

- Feeling abandoned, as they believe that the targeted parent does not love them or care about them, resulting in feelings of anger. Sometimes the anger is extreme, and for some children, the feeling of abandonment impacts on self-esteem as they feel 'unlovable'.
- Feeling angry as a result of being traumatised by the information shared by the alienating parent.
- Learning that relationships are based on conditions and exchanges involving meeting another person's needs to be accepted.
- Learning that their judgement cannot be trusted, since they previously viewed their parent/carer or family member positively.
- Identity or dependency issues, particularly if the alienating parent is enmeshed with the child.
- Difficulties with mentalising, i.e. the ability to see the viewpoint of another, resulting in problems with empathy.
- Being parentified or infantilised, so that the child serves the needs of the alienating parent.
- Low self-esteem and self-worth.
- Poorer performance in school and occupational status.
- Increased vulnerability to mental health issues.
- The behaviours usually impact on the child's relationship with the alienated parent as well as their extended family.
- The extended family of the alienating parent often contributes to or supports the alienating behaviours and therefore puts further pressure on the children to please the alienating parent.

These difficulties can impact on all aspects of a child's social, emotional, cognitive and behavioural functioning and highlight the importance of recognising and attempting to intervene in this insidious form of abuse.

Around 20% of adults who were alienated as children report that they became aware of this when they matured (54), and some have then reunified with the targeted parent (63). This resulted in one-third maintaining a positive, long-term relationship with the targeted parent. There is, however, limited research on the long-term outcomes of alienated children, as most studies have used information provided by adults who say they were exposed to alienating behaviours. Therefore, the frequency and nature of alienating behaviours were not established during childhood and could not be followed up to assess the outcomes.

Conclusions

Parental separation is usually a highly emotional experience for children, even when it is managed sensitively. Children are often asked to take sides in parental disputes and can become embroiled in conflict. Sometimes they believe that one parent has harmed the other and/or themselves. They are often confused about their feelings and can experience torn loyalties, anger, grief and loss. There is significant research to show that the outcome for children following parental separation is significantly better if they continue to maintain relationships with both parents.

If a shared-care arrangement is not possible, then it is important for the child to have regular contact with the non-resident parent and their extended family. In addition, usually children are legally entitled to have access to both parents. It is therefore crucial that if attempts are made by the resident parent to interfere with their relationships with their non-resident parent, professionals should intervene, try to identify difficult behaviours and recommend appropriate support for any child and/or parent in complex circumstances.

References

1   Amato, P.R. (2001). Child of divorce in the 1990s: An update of the Amato and Keith (1991) meta-analysis. *Journal of Family Psychology*, 15, 355–370. doi:10.1037/0893-3200.15.3.355.

2   Amato, P.R. and Anthony, C.J. (2014). Estimating the effects of parental divorce and death with fixed effects models. *Journal of Marriage and Family*, 76, 370–386. doi:10.1111/jomf.12100.

3   Corrás, T., Seijo, D., Fariña, F., Novo, M., Arce, R. and Cabanach, R.G. (2017). What and how much do children lose in academic settings owing to parental separation? *Frontiers in Psychology*. doi:10.3389/fpsyg.2017.01545.

4   Schaan, V.K., Schulz, A., Schächinger, H. and Vögele, C. (2019). Parental divorce is associated with an increased risk to develop mental disorders in women. *Journal of Affective Disorders*, 257, 91–99. doi:10.1016/j.jad.2019.06.071.

5   Seijo, D., Fariña, F., Corrás, T., Novo, M. and Arce, R. (2016). Estimating the epidemiology and quantifying the damages of parental separation in children and adolescents. *Frontiers in Psychology*, 7, 1611. doi:10.3389/fpsyg.2016.01611.

6   Friesen, M.D., Horwood, L.J., Fergusson, D.M. and Woodward, L.J. (2017). Exposure to parental separation in childhood and later parenting quality as an adult: Evidence from a 30-year longitudinal study. *Journal of Child Psychology and Psychiatry*, 58, 30–37. doi:10.1111/jcpp.12610.

7   Vanassche, S., Sodermans, A.K., Declerck, C. and Matthijs, K. (2017). Alternating residence for children after parental separation: Recent findings from Belgium. *Family Court Review*, 55, 545–555. doi:10.1111/fcre.12303.

8   Haux, T. and Platt, L. (2020). Staying involved? The relationship between pre-separation fathering and post-separation contact. *British Politics and Policy at LSE*, 12 August 2020, Blog Entry.

9   Martínez-Pampliega, A., Herrero, M., Cormenzana, S., Corral, S., Sanz, M., Merino, L., Iriarte, L., Ochoa de Alda, I., Alcañiz, L. and Alvarez, I. (2021). Child custody and child symptomatology in high conflict divorce: An analysis of latent profiles. *Psicothema*, 33, 95–102. doi:10.7334/psicothema2020.224.

10 Holt, S. (2016). 'Quality' contact post separation/divorce: A review of the literature. *Child and Youth Services Review*, 68, 92–99. doi:10.1016/j.childyouth.2016.07.001.

11 Cox, R.B., Brosi, M., Spencer, T. and Mosri, K. (2021). Hope, stress and post-divorce child adjustment: Development and evaluation of the co-parenting for resilience

program. *Journal of Divorce and Remarriage*, 62, 144–163. doi:10.1080/10502556. 2021.1871831.

12 Fellmeth, G., Rose-Clarke, K., Zhao, C., et al., (2018). Health impacts of parental migration on left-behind children and adolescents: A systematic review and meta-analysis. *Lancet*, 392, 2567–2582. doi:10.1016/S0140-6736(18)32558-3.

13 Pierce, M., Hope, H.F., Kolade, A., Gellatly, J., Osam, C.S., Perchard, R., Kosidou, K., Dalman, C., Morgan, V., Di Prinzio, P. and Abel, K.M. (2019). Effects of parental mental illness on children's physical health: Systematic review and meta-analysis. *British Journal of Psychiatry*, 271, 354–363. doi:10.1192/bjp.2019.216.

14 Smith, M. (2004). Parental mental health: Disruptions to parenting and outcomes for children. *Child and Family Social Work*. doi:10.1111/j.1365-2206.2004.00312.x.

15 DeVoe, E.R., Ross, A.M., Spencer, R., Drew, A., Acker, M., Paris, R. and Jacoby, V. (2019). Coparenting across the deployment cycle: Observations from military families with young children. *Journal of Family Issues*. doi:10.1177/0192513X19894366.

16 Dunlea, J.P., Wolle, R.G. and Heiphetz, L. (2020). Enduring positivity: Children of incarcerated parents report more positive than negative emotions when thinking about close others. *Journal of Cognition and Development*, 21, 494–512. doi:10.1080/1524 8372.2020.1797749.

17 Bergman, A.S., Axberg, U. and Hanson, E. (2017). When a parent dies – a systematic review of the effects of support programs for parentally bereaved children and their caregivers. *BMC Palliative Care*, 16. doi:10.1186/s12904-017-0223-y.

18 Nickerson, A., Bryant, R.A., Aderka, I.M., Hinton, D.E. and Hofmann, S.G. (2013). The impacts of parental loss and adverse parenting on mental health: Findings from the national comorbidity survey-replication. *Psychological Trauma US*, 5, 119–127. doi:10.1037/A0025695.

19 Thuen, F., Meland, E. and Breidablikk, H.J. (2021). The effects of communication quality and lack of contact with fathers on subjective health complaints and life satisfaction among parental divorced youth. *Journal of Divorce and Remarriage*. doi:10. 1080/10502556.2021.1871835.

20 Kopetski, L. (1998). Identifying cases of parental alienation syndrome – part 1. *The Colorado Lawyer*, 27, 65–68.

21 Dunne, J. and Hedrick, M. (1994). The parental alienation syndrome: An analysis of sixteen selected cases. *Journal of Divorce and Remarriage*, 21, 21–38. doi:10.1300/ J087v21n03_02.

22 Rowan, J. and Emery, R. (2018). Parental denigration: A form of conflict that typically backfires. *Family Court Review*, 56, 258–268.

23 Aloia, L.S. and Strutzenberg, C. (2019). Parent-child communication apprehension: The role of parental alienation and self-esteem. *Communication Reports*, 32, 1–14. doi:10.1080/08934215.2018.1514641.

24 Baker, A.J.L. and Chambers, J. (2011). Adult recall of childhood exposure to parental conflict: Unpacking the black box of parental alienation. *Journal of Divorce and Remarriage*, 52, 55–76. doi:10.1080/10502556.2011.534396.

25 Lang, P.J. (1968). Fear reduction and fear behavior: Problems in treating a construct. In J.M. Shlien (Eds.), *Research in psychotherapy*. Washington, DC: American Psychological Association. doi:10.1037/10546-004.

26 Lang, P.J. (1971). The application of psychophysiological methods to the study of psychotherapy and behavior change. In A.E. Bergin and F.L. Garfield (Eds.), *Handbook of psychotherapy and behavior change: An empirical analysis*. New York: Wiley.

27　Gullone, E. (2000). The development of normal fear: A century of research. *Clinical Psychology Review*, 20, 429–451. doi:10.1016/S0272-7358(99)00034-3.

28　Ollendick, T.H., King, N.J. and Frary, R.B. (1989). Fears in children and adolescents: Reliability and generalisability across gender, age and nationality. *Behaviour Research and Therapy*, 27, 19–26.

29　Muris, P. and Field, A.P. (2010). The role of verbal threat information in the development of childhood fear. "Beware the Jabberwork!" *Clinical Child and Family Psychology Review*, 13, 129–150.

30　Askew, C., Dunne, G., Ösdil, Z., Reynolds, G. and Field, A.P. (2013). Stimulus fear-relevance and the vicarious learning pathway to childhood fears. *Emotion*, 13, 915–925. doi:10.1037/a0032714.

31　Dunne, G. and Askew, C. (2013). Vicarious learning and unlearning of fear in childhood via mother and stranger models. *Emotion*, 13, 974–980. doi:10.1037/a0032994.

32　Rachman, S.J. (1977). The conditioning theory of fear acquisition: A critical examination. *Behaviour Research and Therapy*, 15, 372–387.

33　Marin, M.F., Bilodeau-Houle, A., Morand-Beaulieu, S., Broillard, A., Herringa, S.J. and Milad, M.R. (2020). Vicarious conditioned fear acquisition and extinction in child-parent dyads. *Scientific Reports*, 10.

34　Scarf, D., Gross, J., Colombo, M. and Hayne, H. (2011). To have and to hold: Episode memory in 3–4-year-old children. *Developmental Psychobiology*. doi:10.1002/dev.21004.

35　Gudjonsson, G., Vagni, M., Maiorano, T. and Pajardi, D. (2016). Age and memory related changes in child's immediate and delayed suggestibility using the Gudjonsson suggestibility scale. *Personality and Individual Differences*, 102, 25–29. doi:10.1016/jpaid.2016.06.029.

36　Brewin, C. and Andrews, B. (2017). False memories of childhood abuse. *The Psychologist*, 48–52.

37　Castro, A., Ibáñez, J., Maté, B., Esteban, J. and Barrada, J.R. (2019). Childhood sexual abuse, sexual behaviour and revictimisation in adolescent and youth: A mini review. *Frontiers in Psychology*, 10. doi:10.3389/fpsyg.2019.02018.

38　Papalia, N., Mann, E. and Ogloff, J.R.P. (2020). Child sexual abuse and risk of revictimisation: Impact of child demographics, sexual abuse characteristics and psychiatric disorders. *Child Maltreatment*, 23. doi:10.1177/1077559520932665.

39　Gudjonsson, G.H., Vagni, M., Maiorano, T., Giostra, V. and Pajardi, D. (2021). Trauma symptoms of sexual abuse reduce resilience in children to give 'no' replies to misleading questions. *Personality and Individual Differences*, 168, 1–5. doi:10.1016/jpaid.2020.110378.

40　Gudjonsson, G.H., Vagni, M., Maiorano, T. and Pajardi, D. (2020). The relationship between trauma symptoms and immediate and delayed suggestibility in children who have been sexually abused. *Journal of Investigative Psychology and Offender Profiling*. doi:10.1002/jiip.1554.

41　Raso, C. (2004). *If the bread goes stale, it's my dad's fault: The parental alienation syndrome* (Dissertation). Concordia University, Montreal, Quebec.

42　Warshak, R.A. (2015). Ten parental alienation fallacies that compromise decisions in court and in therapy. *Professional Psychology, Research and Practice*, 46, 235–249.

43　Baker, A.J.L. (2005). The long-term effects of parental alienation on adult children: A qualitative research study. *The American Journal of Family Therapy*, 33, 289–302. doi:10.1080/01926180590962129.

44 Baker, A. and Darnall, D. (2006). Behaviors and strategies employed in parental alienation: A survey of parental experiences. *Journal of Divorce and Remarriage*, 45, 97–104. doi:10.1300/J087v45n01_06.

45 Whitcombe, S. (2017). Parental alienation or justifiable estrangement? Assessing a child's resistance to a parent in the UK. *Seen and Heard*, 27, 1–16.

46 Khaleque, A., Uddin, M.K., Hossain, K.N., Siddique, M.N. and Shirin, A. (2019). Perceived parental acceptance-rejection in childhood predict psychological adjustment and rejection sensitivity in adulthood. *Psychological Studies*, 64, 447–454.

47 Akün, E. (2017). Relations among adults' remembrances of parental acceptance-rejection in childhood, self-reported psychological adjustment, and adult psychopathology. *Comprehensive Psychiatry*, 77, 27–37. doi:10.1016/jcomppsych.2017.05.002.

48 Van Dijk, R., van der Valk, I.E., Deković, M. and Branje, S. (2020). A meta-analysis on interparental conflict, parenting, and child adjustment in divorced families: Examining medication using meta-analytic structural equation models. *Clinical Psychology Review*, 79, 101861. doi:10.1016/j.cpr.2020.101861.

49 Turunen, J., Fransson, E. and Bergström, M. (2017). Self-esteem in children in joint physical custody and other living arrangements. *Public Health*, 149, 106–112. doi:10.1016/jpuhe.2017.04.009.

50 Ben-Ami, N. and Baker, A.J.L. (2012). The long-term correlates of childhood exposure to parental alienation on adult self-sufficiency and well-being. *The American Journal of Family Therapy*, 40, 169–183.

51 Parray, W.M. and Kumar, S. (2017). Impact of assertiveness training on the level of assertiveness, self-esteem, stress, psychological well-being and academic achievement of adolescents. *Indian Journal of Health and Well-Being*, 8, 1476–1480.

52 Khaleque, A. and Rohner, R.P. (2002). Perceived parental acceptance-rejection and psychological adjustment: A meta-analysis of cross-cultural and intracultural studies. *Journal of Marriage and Family*, 64, 54–64. doi:10.1111/j.1741-3737.2002.00054.x.

53 Godbout, E. and Parent, C. (2012). The life paths and lived experiences of adults who have experienced parental alienation: A retrospective study. *Journal of Divorce and Remarriage*, 553, 34–54. doi:10.1080/10502556.2012.635967.

54 Baker, A.J.L. (2007). *Adult children of parental alienation syndrome*. New York: W.W. Norton and Company.

55 Van Dijk, R., van der Valk, I.E., Vossen, H.G.M., Branje, S. and Deković, M. (2021). Problematic internet use in adolescents from divorced families: The role of family factors and adolescents' self-esteem. *The International Journal of Environmental Research and Public Health*, 18, 3385. doi:10.3390/ijerph18073385.

56 Bowlby, J. (1982). Attachment and loss: Retrospect and prospect. *American Journal of Orthopsychiatry*, 52, 664–678. doi:10.1111/j.1939-0025.1982.tb01456.x.

57 Haines, J., Matthewson, M. and Turnbull, M. (2020). *Understanding and managing parental alienation*. Oxon: Routledge.

58 Laughrea, K. (2002). Alienated family relationship scale: Validation with young adults. *Journal of College Student Psychotherapy*, 17. doi:10.1300/J035v17n01_05.

59 Kelly, J.F., Bergman, B., Hoeppner, B.B., Vilsaint, C. and White, W.L. (2017). Prevalence and pathways of recovery from drug and alcohol problems in the United States population: Implications for practice, research and policy. *Drug and Alcohol Dependence*, 162–169.

60 O'Connor, M., Cloney, D., Kvalsvig, A. and Goldfeld, S. (2019). Positive mental health and academic achievement in elementary school: New evidence from a matching analysis. *American Educational Research Association*, 48, 205–216.

61 Agnafors, S., Barmark, M. and Sydsjö, G. (2021). Mental health and academic performance: A study on selection and causation effects from childhood to early adulthood. *Social Psychiatry and Psychiatric Epidemiology*, 56, 857–866.

62 Giofre, D., Borella, E. and Mammarella, I.C. (2017). The relationship between intelligence, working memory, academic self-esteem and academic achievement. *Journal of Cognitive Psychology*, 29. doi:10.1080/20445911.2017.1310110.

63 Darnall, D. and Steinberg, B.F. (2008). Motivational models for spontaneous reunification with the alienated child. Part 1. *American Journal of Family Therapy*, 36, 107–115.

Chapter 8

Typical cases and insights from clinical experience

People who are aware of their behaviours and admit alienation

There are people who are aware and admit they are alienating their children. This does not happen often, but it happens. In my experience the people who have admitted alienating their children have been mothers who alleged their children had been sexually assaulted. I have met people who said they did this for revenge, but mostly mothers who allege the father sexually abused the children, when this did not happen, later say they felt they needed to do this to ensure the father was no longer involved in their children's lives. The alienating parent has tended to blame the targeted parent and struggles to assume responsibility for their own behaviours. To exercise some compassion for the alienating parent, the situation could be understood as a misuse of power in the context of a conflictual relationship which sometimes (but not always) previously had an imbalance of power to the targeted parent. Also, sadly, the alienating parent often has personality issues that do not enable them to demonstrate compassion for their children or the targeted parent. The alienating mothers sometimes say that the father threatened them when they were involved in their relationship with him, they were frightened and that led to the abuse allegations. Alienating fathers say the mothers previously misused their powerful position as the resident parent.

A good outcome

One of the criticisms of parental alienation research is that it involves 'just stories'; however, if this story is yours, then it takes on a different meaning. Some readers might feel I am describing 'stories' below, but it is the case that each individual has a story, and if that story is yours then you want support to try to bring some improvement in functioning to your family. I have attempted to find a balance when talking about the cases. A mother once got annoyed at me for being 'too measured', as she wanted me to agree with her that her husband was a risk to her children, even though she was the one with the significant history of drug use and violence. His history was bumpy, too, but hers had more risk from a parenting point of view.

DOI: 10.4324/9781003156147-8

A good outcome in this context is one where the children are functioning well and there is a resolution in the courts about their future care placements. Sometimes that means moving from the care of the alienating parent, and sometimes it means the targeted parent is unsuccessful in trying to see their children. Whatever is best for the child is the optimum outcome. I know, too, that there are cases that do not have a positive outcome. Professionals have done their best to try to support the family and bring about change, but for a variety of reasons, this does not happen.

Typical cases

The following stories are based on reality but do not apply to any one particular family. As I wanted to ensure anonymity, the reality of the stories is significantly more dramatic than the way I have described them. I asked several parents for comments for the book, and these are also shared. The comments were made anonymously. All the typical cases below result from 'severe' cases of PA (1).

The cases are very loosely based on actual cases from my clinical experience. I have collapsed general themes into stories, and the individuals involved are not identifiable. In my experience, males are as likely to alienate as females if they have the opportunity to do so. The issue often relates to power and control rather than gender. The resident parent is typically the alienating parent, although there are also many cases where the non-resident parent alienated the children whilst they remained in the other parent's care. So from contact one parent persuaded a child to leave the care of the resident parent. The relationship with the resident parent usually ended after this happened. The decision by a child to leave a resident parent typically followed a dispute with them about discipline, for example about tidy bedrooms or internet time. This has happened despite the alienating parent having regular contact with their children without dispute. The confidence to challenge the status quo has sometimes but not always been associated with the arrival of a new partner for either parent. Researchers have also observed alienation by the non-resident parent, and there are findings that particular behaviours are observed in this client group, e.g. encouraging the child to be defiant to the targeted parent, denigrating the targeted parent and oversharing information to encourage parentification of the child so that the child feels they are needed by the alienating parent (1–2).

This is a chapter about typical cases from my clinical practice. They are cases I have seen over a 12-year period. It is only by encountering them that professionals can learn how to prepare and sometimes protect themselves. Without preparation, the professional may feel that they are somehow responsible for the parent's presentation and any heightened emotion that is expressed, i.e. they may feel they are not managing the case well. In my experience, this can easily happen to an unsuspecting professional. Working with this group requires frequent supervision, keeping good notes and making sure the professional person takes good personal care. A clinical psychologist colleague commented that working with alienated parents was like being 'pelted by rocks', and in my experience the alienating parent often turns their anger to the expert. I have had many unpleasant experiences, resulting in my feeling like I needed to lie down in a dark room afterwards. Portrayals of the alienating parent made by some groups as a 'poor person subjected to domestic violence' are not consistent with my experience at all. Although the alienating parent might be vulnerable, they typically express themselves either through charm or high negatively expressed emotion and often vacillate between the two with ease.

There are many publications that describe the prevalence and harm, outcomes, etc., of PA, which provide important background information, but they do not always explain the variability in presentations. Due to a lack of evidence-based research relating specifically to PA interventions, clinicians are limited in the number of management approaches that can be recommended for these complex situations. This is discussed further in the next few chapters. Whilst there have been positive outcomes for some of the cases, many are not resolved, and therefore the child is left to grow up believing the non-resident parent does not love them, and the consequences of this must be considered in any evaluation of the situation. The child also remains in the care of someone who models indifference to the distress they cause others.

Community impact

In small rural communities, untrue allegations of sexual assault are particularly painful for any innocent party if they have been discussed in the community, resulting in a targeted parent being ostracised. They affect not only the person about whom the allegations have been made but also often their extended family, including grandparents and children.

It is difficult to think about how distressed families must feel if a family member has been accused of something that they know is not true, but the community suddenly present as wary and cautious around them, and they are shunned. Sometimes information is shared with teachers or other individuals in the community, who are then obstructive when the accused attempts to attend school productions and/or religious ceremonies. For example, one very experienced teacher I spoke to was particularly negative about a targeted parent when I attempted to discuss the situation with her. Only when the child involved accused another distraught child of sexual assault did the teacher realise that the child did not know the meaning of the words they were using, and the teacher had shunned an ordinary targeted parent and aligned herself with an alienating parent. The teacher was later very apologetic, and the targeted parent was relieved and forgiving. They were all able to move on, but the targeted parent went through a miserable two years beforehand, when they could not attend school events or collect the children because they were perceived in the community as being someone who had sexually assaulted their child.

Therefore, the impact of PA in a small community can be significant and affect many of a targeted parent's relationships, causing unnecessary shame and discomfort.

The age issue

It has been my clinical experience that the older the child is, the more intractable they are when attempts are made to re-engage them in a relationship with their parent. Also, if there are a number of children in a relationship, then typically the eldest stops attending first, and then the next eldest, and so on. Younger children are usually the last to stop attending contact. This is consistent with findings that older and female children are more likely to be alienated than their peers (3).

New partners

New partners are often described by alienating parents as 'father/mother figures', as if a parent can be replaced very easily by a new human. This completely dismisses any emotional connection that a child has to their targeted parent and minimises the role of a parent. It ignores grief and loss that a child might experience when a parent is removed from their lives and indicates to the child that their feelings are not as important as the alienating parent's. Usually the child is expected to have a positive relationship with the new parent irrespective of their level of interest in the child, and there is an assumption that they will like them. Many alienating parents have told me the new parent is 'more of a parent than (the previous parent) will ever be', and they bring their own feelings about the targeted parent to the situation.

Self-harm

Self-harm sometimes occurs when children become overwhelmed by their situation, and they feel they have no other way to communicate their distress. There are occasions when the alienating parent appears pleased that the child is upset, as they blame the targeted parent for any distress felt. This happens even when the child has not seen the targeted parent for many years. I have seen children who bang their heads; cut their arms, legs or tummy; shave their heads and threaten further harm if they are not listened to. This has not changed the behaviour of the alienating parent.

Observations in the home

It has been my experience that even when an alienating parent's home has lots of family pictures, there are none of the targeted parent or their extended family. When I have asked about this, I have been told, 'we're not into family pictures' (despite the 20 or so that I can see), or there are efforts made to distract me. On more than one occasion I have seen children run back to the alienating parent and whisper loudly (because sometimes when they are young, they forget how to be discreet) and ask the alienating parent to remind them what they are supposed to say.

The voice of the child

On many occasions, when I have seen children without the alienating parent, they have asked me not to repeat or write down what they are saying. Many have asked me to read aloud what I have written about the interview and asked me to write down what they were told to say, as opposed to what they really think. Therefore, the voice of the child is not really heard, if they can only share information that they have been given to say.

Allegations of sexual assault of the child

Many cases involve allegations of sexual assault of the child. This usually follows if other attempts to end contact have not been successful. Sometimes the child does not know the allegation has been made, but on other occasions this involves the child going through detailed social worker and police interviews and intimate examinations at a centre for those who have been sexually assaulted. It has been my experience that even after these events produce no suggestion or evidence of sexual assault, the alienating parent will continue to claim that this has occurred. Professionals are aware that not all sexual assaults leave physical evidence, and sometimes later the allegations are retracted, although the incidence of this is low. Even when retracted the alienating parent will say, 'I retracted them because I had no choice. I still believe that they were sexually assaulted', or they will vacillate between thinking the child might have been assaulted and saying they made it up because they felt threatened by the situation.

Secret recordings

I have been secretly and not-so-secretly recorded many times now. Sometimes this has involved a mobile phone on the table recording what is being said (I usually spot this and ask about it; often the person recording puts the phone away then), but there have also been video recordings. One of the solicitors told me they listened to a 'long and boring four hours' of voice recording, which was entirely consistent with the report. One professional person rang me from court saying that the alienating parent said he had recorded the session and was going to the newspapers. I assume the newspapers did not feel this was really a story of interest, as I never heard anything more about it. One of the video recordings was apparently stolen from one parent and given to the other parent by a child involved in the conflict. The purpose of the recordings appeared to be an effort to undermine the psychological assessment, and it is important for professionals involved to be aware that this can happen and to be able to stand over everything they have said.

Case study 1 – admission of lies

In one of my early cases, a very assertive, high-functioning woman who held a professional job told me she had been seriously sexually assaulted on a first date with her future husband. She had then gone on to have three children with him. Although her GP notes and records reflected stability, with reports of the father being supportive for many years, once the couple separated, the mother reported that during the relationship, she had experienced sustained physical aggression including repeated sexual assault. It can happen that the medical records note a stable background whilst there is control or disturbance in the relationship, particularly as it begins to break down. The mother and father and children were all high-functioning, with no signs of any mental health difficulties or vulnerabilities likely to be associated with living in a home where violence was regularly taking place (although some children cope incredibly well with a high level of violence in the home).

It was then reported that the children did not want to see the father, and a year later it was said that he had sexually assaulted one of them. I saw this particular child for assessment, and in the presence of the mother, I very carefully began to allude to the allegations. The mother looked horrified, and the child clearly had no idea what I was talking about, so I did not pursue it. I saw the mother again on a different day, and she was alone. I reflected again on her experiences, giving her the opportunity to raise any issues, as it appeared the child was unaware of the assault allegations. The mother started to cry and said she had made it all up. Her husband had been loving and caring and had never been aggressive, but she had met a new partner and did not want the father to be part of her children's lives any longer. When I spoke to the father on the phone, he was demanding and overbearing, and I was reminded of a legal professional's comment about alienating mothers, who said 'it's all they have', referring to women who use parental alienation to harm their ex-partners. This was their explanation of the reasoning behind the behaviour rather than condoning it.

Outcome

In this case the children remained in the care of their mother, and they stopped seeing their father.

Case study 2 – allegations of sexual abuse in a small community

In this case the father worked away a lot and the mother remained at home. Both parents alleged the other had been unfaithful. It seemed that, like a lot of couples, they simply drifted apart, with the father working away from home a lot and focused on earning money. He felt that he had everything he wanted. Meanwhile the mother was focused on childcare and keeping the home, although she felt lonely and dissatisfied. During the marriage breakdown (at which time parents are typically not at their best), the parents both drank more alcohol than they usually did, and they went through a period of separation followed by reconciliation, only to result in arguments again. They finally separated after allegations of domestic violence. One incident was particularly salient, when one parent locked the other out of the home (they both agreed on this part of the story) after a violent incident when they squirted each other with tomato ketchup and other foods. However, both parties did not agree with the allegation that one party had threatened to harm the other with a screwdriver. There were no physical injuries. What was particularly interesting was that the description of the screwdriver changed frequently, as did the story about the context in which it happened, which led to some suspicion about the reliability of the allegations.

The couple separated. Neither had a mental health history, and there were no other reports of violence. The father was close to his family and lived with them when the relationship ended. The mother remained in the family home with the children.

Within a few months, the eldest girl stopped attending contact, then the next child, and so on, until the contact stopped. The children said their father had attacked their mother with a screwdriver. Detail about the incident varied. The mother accused the father of domestic violence, and after about six months or so of court intervention, trying to reintroduce the children to their father, the mother also alleged sexual assault of the youngest children. When the mother reported this to the professionals involved, the youngest children supported her assertions, although the police felt the reports were unusual. The case confused everyone involved because the children frequently changed their accounts about what exactly had happened. When the case proceeded through the courts, the mother increased her efforts to exclude the father from the children, telling other parents in the school yard that he was a paedophile and calling this out to him when she saw him. The father, worried about what others in the community thought, avoided people for many years. His family supported him, and they too avoided community events.

Many assessments were carried out by professionals, and the courts looked widely for appropriate experts. During my assessment the mother was adamant that the children had been sexually assaulted, although she would tell me about this whilst rather unusually smiling at the same time. In addition, she was evasive throughout the assessment and minimised any issues that might arise from the children believing they had been sexually assaulted if this were not true. She appeared to find the process entertaining rather than distressing, and she did not appear to be emotionally connected with the material that we were discussing.

After hearing all the evidence, the court delivered its conclusion, and I was asked to engage with the children therapeutically. Part of my role was to identify the implications for the children of having to say they had been sexually assaulted if this had not taken place and try to ameliorate any harm resulting from this. In advance of this meeting, I saw the mother to discuss what the session would involve. I saw the children together with their mother, and other professionals observed. To make the session child-friendly and to allow the children to forgive their mother, I explained that their parents had a disagreement and their mother had said something that she regretted because it was not true (whether she regretted it is debatable; however, she was listening and did not intervene). I said that it seemed their father may not have touched their 'bottoms'; this was simply something mummy had said when she was cross. One child (aged five years) said nothing and simply nodded, as if they knew this was some sort of adult issue in which they were not getting involved. The second child (aged seven years) said, 'I wondered. I knew I couldn't remember it. I thought it must have happened when I was asleep'. The children had previously told many professionals that the father had sexually assaulted them and yet remained uncertain about whether or how it had happened.

Subsequently, significant efforts were made to engage the mother with professionals, including an offer of psychological intervention. The mother remained unremorseful and adamant the children should not see their father. Unusually in these cases, she admitted that she had made up the stories about abuse because she wanted revenge on her husband for past behaviours. She said he had been violent towards her, and when I explored this fully, it seemed that they had behaved poorly towards each other, although the father had the potential to be significantly more threatening than the mother due to his physicality. Finally, I had a meeting with both parents. The father presented as reasonable and said, 'Why did this happen?' The mother smiled at him and did not respond. I said, 'I was told this morning that this was about revenge'. The father said, 'Is it over now, has she got revenge?' I looked at the smiling mother, and when it was clear she did not intend to respond, I said, 'Sadly, I don't think so'. The mother did not contradict me. The father sighed and then said, 'I haven't seen John for a long time. Does he still like sailing?' The mother said, 'Not anymore. He likes skateboarding now', before looking at me quickly. As I had spoken to John the previous evening, I was aware he remained as passionate as ever about sailing. I said, 'Yes, John still likes sailing'. The mother looked at me and smiled.

In this case, significant efforts were made to re-start contact with the father whilst the children remained in the mother's care, but these were mostly unsuccessful. There were some positive meetings with the extended family, particularly a previously much-loved aunt; however, the children protested to any suggestion they would meet their father. After some time working towards building up a relationship with the aunt, who was seen independently, it was decided that the father would join the contact. No professionals were present for this, although a trusting relationship had been developed with the aunt. The children were reported to have been wary of the father, but nothing untoward was reported, and gradually the father spent a little bit more time each week with the children. One day a professional person rang me to say she had just parked her car outside the aunt's home, and the children had not seen her, but they were playing in the garden with the father. She said they were shrieking with laughter.

Sadly, although the children were clearly enjoying their relationship with their father again, each time they returned to the care of the mother, they said they did not want to see their father, as he had 'held a screwdriver' to the mother's throat. This story became more dramatic over time, and the children presented as uncomfortable and distressed when they told it. The relationships between the father and his children were slowly building, but they did not resolve their situation whilst they lived with the mother.

Outcome

The children were eventually removed to the care of the extended family and finally the father. One year later I visited them in school to see how they were functioning. The children presented as happy, and the principal of the school told me he was surprised by how quickly the children's presentation changed when they moved to the father's care. He described them as more engaged with their education and with extracurricular events. He felt they had been weighed down by the conflict between their parents and were eventually freed up to enjoy their lives when they went to their father's care.

Some years later when I contacted the father (and received his permission to include his story in this book), he had continued to support the children's relationship with their mother, and they were dropped off once or twice a week to see her under supervision by the mother's extended family. Apparently the children found the contact difficult at times, as they were met with a high level of criticism from the mother about their appearance, but they were happy to see her, and they loved her and her extended family. The father reassured them about their appearance when they returned to his care and felt they recovered quickly from any negative comments made.

When I was thinking about this book, I asked the father what would he say to others in a similar situation, and he told me, 'Tell the truth. The entire story. If you focus on the truth, everyone will find out what really happened'.

Case study 3 – child self-harm

The parents were involved in a relationship for over 20 years and had five children, aged five to 15 years old. The children were close to both sets of grandparents. The mother was a 'homemaker', and the father worked in his family's business. The mother was happy and said she did not realise the father was becoming disgruntled with the relationship.

In this case the mother said that the father ended the relationship without warning. Also, because he owned the home before he met the mother, he said this justified his asking the mother and children to move out of the family residence. The mother did as she was asked, and the children moved to another home with her. They had regular contact with the father, although it seemed that the mother was controlling at times and critical of the father. Unfortunately, the mother did not cope well with her new situation, and when one of the children reported she was smacking as a means of managing behaviour, the children were removed from the mother's care and placed with the father. Interestingly, when I spoke to the children, they reported that both parents had previously used smacking occasionally as a form of punishment.

Difficulties emerged when the mother attempted to have contact with the children, and the father sent unhelpful and hurtful text messages to the mother telling her that the children did not want to see her. The children were court-ordered to attend supervised contact with the mother but often arrived, said they did not want to attend and walked away.

The stress the children experienced began to emerge, and one female child and one male child began to present with signs and symptoms of a physical response to emotional difficulties. They had headaches, tummy aches, etc., for which no physical cause was found. It was noted that when the children did not attend contact, the father was offering them a more attractive alternative, i.e. shopping for game consoles, make-up, etc. This issue was drawn to the attention of the father, who denied these allegations. The case was referred for assessment. When the medical records were reviewed, it was clear the children were experiencing stress resulting from their situation, which the father said was a consequence of the history with the mother. The thing is, the children did not attend their GP complaining of stress when they lived with both parents, and it seemed that the children's experience of being involved in the parents' conflict was causing them significant levels of anxiety, rather than contact per se.

When I spoke to the mother, she recognised that her behaviour towards the children had been poor during the relationship breakdown and said that she been inconsolable with grief and not managed herself very well during this time. She admitted smacking them but denied that she had assaulted them beforehand.

The children were observed having contact with their mother in a local park, although the two eldest children would not agree to attend, saying they 'just didn't want to go'. The next eldest child hung back before leaving her father, looking at him for permission to leave. The father looked at me intensely and did not look at the child, so the girl said, 'Where are you going to?' and the father, aware he had been accused of offering preferable alternatives to contact, said, 'I'm just going for a drive'. The girl said, 'Well, I'll just go for a walk then', and she looked as if she was not sure whether she should leave or not. I said, 'Let's go', and the girl came with me and the other two children.

The youngest two children ran to the mother, wanted to be close to her, were highly excited about the contact and asked to sit next to her when they stopped their walk for a picnic. The girl who had expressed hesitation slowly engaged with the mother, and although she initially hung back, over time she moved closer to her and attempted to gain the mother's attention frequently, so that if one child did something that the mother commented on, this girl then repeated the action. The children, particularly the child who was initially reticent, asked me on many occasions what time it was and expressed sadness about how quickly the time with their mother was going. They walked back to their father in silence, and I thanked the father for allowing them to see their mother, hoping that he might see that by allowing them contact he had been generous and given his children some relief from the stress they experienced from the parental difficulties.

Sadly, this case continued, and the emotional welfare of the girl who was caught in her parents' conflict deteriorated. During one contact session she arrived having just shaved her head. The supervisors reported the issue, saying that on that occasion when the girl came to contact, she cried constantly. She asked the supervisors to help her, saying she wanted to please both her parents, but she could not do this as one parent wanted her to attend contact and the other did not.

Outcome

In this case all the children were harmed by their experiences. The extent of harm related to the children's relationships with their parents and siblings, their self-esteem and their level of resilience. Most children who love both their parents are likely to be distressed if they feel they cannot meet both their needs. In this case the two youngest children were excited about seeing the mother and ignored the father's subtle attempts to persuade them to stay, and the two eldest were alienated by the father and expressed anger towards the mother. One child was caught in the middle. Most alienating parents that I meet seem to hope to quash the love the child has for the other parent, not responding to any suggestions that this might be harmful for the child.

Case study 4 – removal to the care of the targeted parent

A father believed the couple was happy until he discovered the mother was having an affair, and she ended the relationship. The children were reported to have had a close relationship with their father and paternal grandmother, even after the parents' relationship ended. The father supported the mother by taking the children when she needed him to, if she had work or other commitments. This worked well for a year or so. The mother met a new partner, and the father suddenly found that he was no longer needed for childcare. The mother started to say that the children, then aged three, four and five, no longer wanted to see their father. The father looked for professional help, and with the court's support, a schedule for contract was drawn up. The children then either did not appear for contact or turned up crying and saying they did not want to see their father, and on these occasions, not wanting to cause them further distress, he went home without seeing them. One day, the father was shocked to receive a phone call saying that he had been accused of sexually assaulting his daughter during their most recent contact. For a couple of years, the father did not see the children, and he described his devastation about the allegations. He was also extremely upset when he learned about the intimate examinations his children had to go through. One day his four-year-old daughter went into school and said one of the other children in her class had sexually assaulted her. The teacher knew that there had been no opportunity for this to occur and reported the incident to social work professionals.

When I saw the father, he was distraught about what had happened. An arrangement was made in court for the mother to bring the children to see me at my offices, with an understanding that they would meet the father. The date for meeting the father was not specified. After speaking to the children about their father and showing them some pictures of him (there was no distress when they saw the pictures), I suggested during the session that we would bring the father in. The mother agreed, and I texted the father, who was happy to comply, and he arrived shortly afterwards at my office. The mother then behaved as though she needed to protect the children, and they quite suddenly presented as terrified of him, scrambling around the mother and trying to climb on top of her. The father attempted to reach out to the mother, suggesting they put their experiences behind them and prioritise the children's needs. In the presence of the children, the mother shouted at the father, calling him names and saying he had physically assaulted all of them and sexually assaulted his daughter. The mother walked out of the office, holding two of the children's hands, whilst they held their heads low and kept their backs to their father. Sadly, after they left the room, the father asked me if I would mind if he looked out the window at them, as it had been so long since he had last seen them. He appeared despondent but then contained his emotions and focused on talking about his situation.

A short time after the clinical psychology report was submitted, a professional person brought the children to see their father without the mother present. It seemed the absence of the mother was key in this case. The father brought their favourite toys from when they spent time with him. They initially hung back, but after some hesitation they began to engage with him again, and by the time the one hour of contact ended, they presented as comfortable and settled in his care. Two further similar sessions were observed by professionals, during which time the children were excited to see the father and ran towards him as soon as they saw him. They were affectionate and relaxed in his company. The children presented as more comfortable with the father than with the mother and were temporarily placed in the care of their father, whilst the mother completed an intervention, and it was suggested a shared-care arrangement could be introduced in the future.

Outcome

After the children were removed to the care of the father, it was recommended that the mother engage in a programme of therapeutic work, whilst the children had supervised contact with her. The intention was that the children would have a shared-care arrangement with their parents once the mother engaged with professionals. This appeared to be an excellent approach, suggested by legal professionals, and offered the mother an opportunity to re-engage as a parent. Interestingly, the mother did not want to engage with professionals, even when it was court ordered and she had been informed her children would not be returned to her care unless she did so.

Subsequently, one year later, the children presented as more settled in preschool and school and had all won prizes for their work and behaviour since moving to the care of the father. The mother's attendance at contact was intermittent. She continued to refuse to engage in any therapeutic intervention. Separately, I saw the children with both parents on several occasions, and they presented as significantly more confident, happy and engaged with the father. The mother was critical of the children when she was with them, and when I asked her about this, she appeared to lack awareness of her behaviours. She appeared to lack empathy for the children and her ex-partner, although she acknowledged that her ex-partner had been successful in parenting the children and said she 'got confused' when she alleged sexual assault. However, within a very short period of time she changed her opinion and vacillated between claiming the allegations were real and then expressing regret and sorrow and saying she did not mean them. It was difficult to know what she really thought.

This case indicated that no matter how much help is offered to some parents, they will not engage in intervention, and although a path for reunification was clear for the mother, she was not interested in doing this, even for the benefit of the children. The mother demonstrated that she could not prioritise the children's need to see her above her own needs, and what they are remains to be identified. This does not mean the approach would not be helpful for all parents, as I have seen it used with other families more successfully.

Case study 5 – resident parent becomes targeted parent

The parents were together for around five years and had three children, two boys and one girl. The father was a professional person. The mother had some temporary part-time employment at times, although her main role was looking after her children. The parents separated, and the mother later alleged that the father was violent and controlling throughout their relationship. The father said the mother was generally unhappy and disengaged. Despite their differences, for nine years contact took place regularly, without issue from the mother's perspective, although the father would say that the mother was 'controlling' about the pick-up times, etc.

The mother met a new partner, and the children were reported to have good relationships with him and their two younger half-siblings. One day the mother had an argument with the eldest boy from her first marriage, who was then aged 14 years. She told me he ran out of their home and contacted the father, who arrived shortly afterwards and collected him. The father had recently become engaged to a new partner. The boy did not return to the mother's care, and she initially believed that some time with his father might be helpful to him and did not pursue reconciliation. The other two children continued to see their father at the weekends as usual.

One evening on their return from contact on a Sunday evening, the remaining two children were very quiet. They ran upstairs to prepare for the week ahead as usual whilst the mother served dinner. Without the mother's knowledge, they went to their bedrooms and packed their clothes. The father was waiting for them outside the home, and they walked out past their mother with their belongings. The mother was distraught and begged the children to stay.

Subsequently, the children did not have contact with the mother. Attempts at family therapy were unsuccessful, and every time a glimmer of success was evident, the father quashed it. The children were reported to be distraught during family therapy, and the father blamed the mother for their distress. During sessions the children used adult language to describe their experiences with their mother. The mother said she did not recognise the account they gave of her parenting, and the family therapist said the children clearly wanted to change the situation with their mother, but the father controlled the sessions. When the children showed signs of softening their stance towards the mother, the father interjected and eventually removed them from therapy altogether, saying it was too hard for them and he did not wish to subject them to it. The father would not permit the children to be seen without him. His partner was with him at all the family therapy sessions.

When I saw the father, he said he did not feel the children needed to see their mother as he had a new partner who was 'more of a mother than she has ever been'. It seemed to me that the new partner was influential with the father and had decided not to permit the children to see their mother. After some discussion about the negative impact of the children not having a relationship with their mother, the father seemed to consider the prospect of contact. I suggested that the children could meet the mother for coffee in a city centre. He could be in the area in case there were any complications or concerns, and they all had mobile phones. Sadly, although he agreed to this when I was with him, the meeting did not materialise, and the children stopped seeing their mother altogether.

Outcome

It is my understanding the children have two other siblings that they have not met, and they did not see their mother again.

Case study 6 – an arrest

This case involved parents who went to school together. They dated and married at a very young age, although the father said he was never totally sure this was what he wanted to do and was swept along by the mother's enthusiasm. After the couple was married, they both felt unhappy, and the mother expressed concerns about her sexuality. The father supported the mother to have same-sex relationships, and they both decided that they had married too young and should separate. The father's emotional welfare began to deteriorate, although he had good family support, and after a period of grieving his functioning improved again. His mother and father lived nearby, and the father came and went from the children's home, providing afterschool care and taking the children some weekends with flexibility for both the parents and the children. For some time, this arrangement worked well, and the children and parents were all settled with their arrangement.

Both sets of grandparents were also very involved and provided childcare when both parents were unavailable. The parents had two children, one girl and one boy.

One night when the father and children were watching a film together, the police came to the home and took him in for questioning associated with sexually assaulting his children. The father was devastated that the children saw him leave the family home in a police car. The arresting police officer was kind, and the father was quickly released without charge.

The father was told the children did not want to see him again, and contact stopped. The father took the case before the court, and contact was granted. Supervised contact began, albeit with difficulty, as the mother turned up with the children and waited for them, and the children tended to run back to her. I observed contact several times, and the children were angry and rude to the father. They called him by his first name and told him he had been aggressive towards their mother. They accused him of 'kicking' and 'punching' the mother and calling her names. Although I did not hear either parent use swear words, the children used language that was shocking, given their ages (five and six years). The father was calm and responded as best anyone could to these allegations. He attempted to appeal to the children in a range of ways, using distraction and attempting to have some quality time with them. He was gentle but did not permit the children to mistreat him, and at times he firmly reminded them that they used to enjoy being with him. The younger child appeared to be interested in getting to know him and when separated from the sibling could enjoy time with the father. The elder child appeared to be determined that no 'fun time' would take place and constantly interrupted the father's contact with the sibling, even when a supervising professional asked them not to. Oddly, when the father offered the elder child some favourite sweets, these were accepted without looking at him, and I saw her touch his hand affectionately, whilst at the same time delivering a tirade of abuse. The mother arrived late for contact and waited for a while, and then she turned up early to collect the children. She presented as bright and breezy and confident, with no concerns about the children's unusual presentation, and she happily walked alongside the father, chatting to him about the environment.

Outcome

When I last heard about this case the father continued to try to see his children, and the contact sessions were irregular and interrupted by the mother's unpredictable attendance. The children continued to say they did not wish to attend.

Case study 7 – targeted grandparents

I also observed a contact session with some paternal grandparents who had previously looked after three children whilst the mother worked. The paternal grandparents were reported to have been very close to the children, and there were many pictures to suggest affectionate and happy relationships. The grandparents were confused and distraught about their situation. Before contact took place, a meeting was held between social services staff and the mother to ensure everyone was clear about what would happen. I was not present for this meeting, but I was made aware that the arrangement was for the grandparents to take the children for ice-cream. On the day of contact I happened to arrive early and parked my car. I saw the mother calmly walk across the car park, returning shortly afterwards with the children, who were eating ice-cream. When the mother arrived with the children to meet the grandparents for the one-hour contact session, they held ice-creams in their hands. It was clear that the arrangement was not going to proceed as planned. The mother then immediately said she needed to take the children back to the car to get their coats. Fortunately, there was also a social worker present, and she returned to the mother's car with her to collect coats whilst I proceeded with the children and grandparents to the contact session. When the social worker got to the car with the mother, the coats were not in it, and it turned out the children already had their coats in their backpacks with them.

The grandparents had brought gifts, and the youngest child showed some signs of shifting towards engagement with the contact session; however, the eldest child was determined to disrupt this, and the grandparents said nothing when the eldest child was extremely rude and disparaged their gifts, adding that they had mistreated their mother. The eldest child used vulgar and disturbing language. Towards the end of contact, during a brief settled period, the children and grandparents managed to have a brief positive exchange before the mother arrived with histrionic presentation. I asked the eldest child if we could discuss some of the allegations she had made about the grandparents with her mother, but the child said she could no longer remember them and she wanted to go home.

Outcome

The children never saw their grandparents again.

Case study 8 – when people lose their way

The case involved two parents, both in high-profile jobs, both with access to other people's children. They also had a business, which was very profitable, and they had homes in four different countries. They led a modest life to most people who knew them. The couple both seemed to revel in the contradictions of their life, and it seemed that for many years, this worked well for them. One male child was born from this relationship.

Towards the end of their relationship, not unusually, squabbling took place between the parties. According to the mother, the child was manipulated by the father throughout the marriage, and the father said the child just favoured his company. As the relationship deteriorated, it seemed the mother managed her situation by withdrawing and remaining distant, and the father described her as 'cold'. The parents then accused each other of having affairs, and it seemed they had both had relationships with other people. The father claimed his affair was brief, and the mother reported she did not get involved with anyone else until after the relationship had ended. The couple separated and the boy remained with the mother, although from her account the relationship was strained. The father then began to make the mother's life extremely uncomfortable by behaving bizarrely. On one occasion, the mother said she came home to find that her home had been broken into, and her bed was 'decorated' with many personal items of an intimate nature. Pictures were taken and left on the bed with a note to say these would be sent to mutual friends if she did not agree to permit the son to live with his father.

When the mother responded angrily, the father cried during his next contact with the son. He gained the support of the child, and the mother was seen as the 'bad parent' who had caused distress. It seemed that the father used the contact sessions to manipulate the child, persuading him that the mother was not to be trusted. The child brought the father's arguments back to the home and presented as angry and irritable with her. The mother struggled to manage the situation and withdrew even more.

Family therapy was attempted on several occasions by highly experienced family therapists; however, the father was reported to constantly manipulate the sessions, and eventually therapists concluded they could not proceed. Both parents attempted to manipulate their psychological assessment, which was completed after family therapy had been attempted on at least two occasions by different therapists.

Outcome

Subsequently after one particular contact session, the boy refused to return to the care of his mother. By that time, the boy was not seeing his maternal family at all. A maternal grandparent he had previously been very close to died, and he did not attend the funeral. The child remained in the care of the father, and the mother stopped seeing him.

Case study 9 – retaliation for domestic violence

The father and mother had three children, all girls. The mother alleged the father was jealous of her relationships with other males throughout their time together, and it appeared that there was a certain level at which the mother enjoyed this attention. There were indications that the mother exploited the father's insecurities by flirting with male friends and telling him that other men were interested in her. The father had many friends who frequently visited the home, and the father said the mother was disparaging of his relationship with them, claiming they had visited to see her. In support of this, the mother told me the same thing. The relationship deteriorated, although neither parent wanted to end the relationship at that time.

One evening the mother went out with friends, and the father was at home with the children. The father thought the mother looked beautiful when she left the home, and after she left, he began to feel upset. He thought she did not dress up so nicely when she went out with him, and he began to wonder whether she was having an affair. The father texted the mother all evening, receiving either abrupt or no responses. By the time the mother returned home, quite intoxicated, in the early hours of the following morning, the father was waiting for her. The father assaulted the mother, hitting her and pulling her hair, before leaving the family home. Shortly before he left, the children woke up and, hearing the commotion, came into the living area to see their father hurting their mother. The mother described a high level of fear, and she presented as traumatised by what happened. No one ever denied that the level of violence was atrocious, including the father, who apologised many times. He was aware that an apology did not remove the incident or change the impact it had on his family.

The father left the family home and admitted what he had done to the police. He had no history of violence or any untoward behaviour. He regretted his actions and told the mother he was sorry. He presented as very remorseful but remained adamant that the mother had been having an affair. He knew, however, that whether she had been having an affair or not, his behaviour had been completely inappropriate.

The children had some contact with the father, with mixed success. Over time, it was reported they did not want to attend. The courts became involved, and a psychological assessment was instructed. The mother told me the father was going to 'kill' the children, and so they could not attend contact. The mother demonstrated signs and symptoms of an emotional response to a traumatic event, and she completed trauma-focused Cognitive Behavioural Therapy (as per the NICE guidelines at that time). During this time, it became clear that the mother did not respond to therapeutic intervention, and she continued to say the father would 'kill' the children if he saw them.

Due to the mother's allegations that the father would hurt the children, a senior social worker got involved with the case and tried to help the father by supervising contact twice a week for four months. The social worker said the contact was of a high quality, and the children clearly benefited a great deal from it. Each week the children became a little less wary of the father, until they were clearly excited to see him, hugged him spontaneously and spoke enthusiastically about him. Eventually, the social worker had to withdraw from the supervision, and at that time, there were no concerns about the father's ability to parent the children appropriately or about them presenting as frightened of him. In fact, it was reported they presented as excited and jumped on him when they saw him, and at the end of each contact, they planned the next one.

Outcome

The next time I heard about this case, the mother had immediately stopped the children from seeing the father once the social worker withdrew. The father was powerless and had given up trying to have a relationship with his children.

Case study 10 – alienating a family

This was a particularly sad case. The mother met the father on holiday abroad, where he had a summer job as a casual labourer. The mother came home after a summer 'fling' and found she was pregnant. She contacted the father, they remained in contact, and after the child was born, they visited each other annually. The father did not have a positive relationship with the mother or her family, and visits were fraught with tension. The father wanted the child to have a different name and a different religion and presented as unhappy with the mother's liberal culture and approach to parenting.

The mother's family supported her at a high level, and she and the child lived with a maternal uncle, who was referred to as 'dad'. The biological father was known as 'papa'. Dad was very involved in the child's care, made breakfast, took the child to and from school each day, and provided afterschool care until the mother returned from work. Sadly, the mother was involved in a road traffic accident and died at the scene. Dad and the child were waiting for her to return from work. The biological father was contacted, and when he arrived, he immediately asserted himself and his role. There appeared to be very little consideration about the impact of events on the child. The child moved to the care of the father, and promises were made about how the child would be raised, including the fact that the child would remain at the same school and maintain relationships with their maternal family.

Outcome

I saw the child ten years after I originally met the family. When I met the child the second time, they had a different name and a new religion. They had moved to a new area and had no contact with their maternal family. They refused to talk about 'dad', although they were able to speak enthusiastically about their new 'mum' and about their biological father's family.

Case study 11 – a private detective

The parents both worked in professional jobs and had two children. There had been some domestic violence before the relationship ended, and they both admitted pushing each other and kicking. It seemed that no one parent was more guilty than the other of violence.

The parents decided to separate and had a joint-care arrangement. One day when the father returned the children to the mother, she alleged he had called her names in front of the children, and she therefore refused to permit them to see him again. The father went to court, and because he had dashcam he had inadvertently recorded the handover, without either him or the mother knowing. He discovered this some time after the allegations were made. This enabled him to demonstrate to the court that he had not been aggressive, and shared care resumed. Shortly after this, the mother alleged that the father had hit one of the children. The child was not taken to the family doctor, and there were no bruises or marks, but to ensure their safety, the father's contact with the children was supervised for some time, gradually returning to a shared-care arrangement. Both parents met new partners, although their battle in court continued. The mother left her employment but did not disclose this fact to the court and said her children needed to attend a school near where she worked so that she could be available for them. The location of the school made it difficult for the father to collect them, but he continued to try to do this. On the days when the father was not available, he hoped that the paternal grandparents would be able to get involved, but the mother did not permit this. The mother asserted that the children should always be collected by her after school, no matter whether the father was available or not.

Outcome

The court decided that the father could collect his children from school. The mother hired a private detective to ensure that the father was doing this. The private investigator followed the father to the children's school, then watched him strap them into their seats and take them to the paternal grandparents' home. The mother then went back to court and stated the father should not have the children because they were not consistently in his care. The father had not actually done anything that the mother could complain about, but she continued to complain that she was sure he would harm them. Fortunately for the father, one of the concerns that the mother had was that social workers were involved in her life and she did not want her neighbours to know this. This led to her agreeing that the father could see the children again without social worker intervention. This resulted in an arrangement whereby the father had regular contact with the children, who remained in the care of the mother.

Case study 12 – grandiosity

The mother in this case was grandiose and the father quiet and unassertive. The mother had children by three different fathers, none of whom had contact. Each father appeared to assume the bulk of the chores in the family, including childcare, and when they were unavailable, other family members stepped in. The mother was perceived to have a physical health condition, but the medical notes revealed a psychosomatic disorder. The mother alleged inappropriate gifts were given, and the children supported this assertion. For example, the mother said the children had been given gifts that were likely to cause her distress, as they suggested that she was not parenting appropriately, even though the gifts were innocuous, i.e. pyjamas, slippers, vouchers, etc.

The children would not engage with professionals and were reported to be mute when attempts were made to interview them. I was told they had no positive memories of their history with their father and could not remember their paternal extended family. When I saw them separately from the mother and out of earshot, they were funny and engaging and remembered fun times with their extended family. When I showed them pictures of themselves with the father, they laughed and were able to add information to the pictures. Next time I met them, they were with the mother and suddenly they were mute again. The mother stood between them and me, as if to protect them. In the presence of the mother, they would not agree to see the father.

Outcome

The child did not see the father again.

Case study 13 – new sibling

The children lived with the mother after the parents separated, and the youngest child was born after the father left the family home. For many years the children had contact with the father until the mother met a new partner, and suddenly the children no longer wanted to see him and they reported to 'idolise' their new 'daddy'. The father attempted to persuade the mother to change her mind about contact, and this was unsuccessful, so he went to court to see if this would help.

The mother was entrenched in her position, as was her extended family. During the court process, one contact between the father's new daughter, who was a toddler, and the children was arranged. The children clearly loved seeing their half-sibling, were very excited during the session and asked me to take many pictures of them. I was able to share these pictures with the father, who sadly was unable to see the children himself.

Outcome

Unfortunately, the mother did not permit any further contact, and no further court intervention took place.

Conclusion

Although these cases might be described as 'just stories', they are based on real cases. In my clinical experience it is usually the resident parent who stops contact, but resident parent/child relationships can be harmed during contact sessions, and a child can be alienated from their parent during this time. The children's emotional welfare seems not to matter to the alienating parent, which makes these cases extremely sad. These cases are muddled up and changed, and although I may have lost some of the detail in the translation, as each study is based on more than one case, the reality is that accurate descriptions of the cases would make them seem much more unlikely than the situations presented here.

References

1   Warshak, R.A. (2013). Severe cases of parental alienation. In D. Lorendos, W. Bernet and S.R. Sauber (Eds.), *American series in behavioural science and law: Parental alienation: The handbook for mental health and legal professionals* (pp. 74–96). Springfield, IL: Charles C. Thomas Publisher.
2   López, T.J., Iglesias, V.E.N. and García, P.F. (2014). Parental alienation gradient: Strategies for a syndrome. *The American Journal of Family Therapy*, 42, 217–231. doi:10.1080/01926187.2013.820116.
3   Baker, A.J.L. and Darnell, D. (2008). Behaviors and strategies employed in parental alienation. *Journal of Divorce and Remarriage*. doi:10.1300/J087v45n01_06.

Chapter 9

The assessment

Introduction

There may be years of protracted proceedings before a case reaches clinical psychology for assessment. Typically, the targeted parent, who cannot gain access to their child, seeks legal advice. There is often a period of months or years before this, where the targeted parent is working hard towards seeing their children and has contact with them intermittently, before they finally give up and seek help from legal services. Often the alienating parent says that the child will attend contact if the targeted parent stops proceedings, and sometimes they stop, only to find they do not see their child as agreed. As the process in court can take time, this sometimes results in the targeted parent not seeing the child for a very long time. This period without contact is then sometimes used against the targeted parent as 'proof' that they did not try to gain contact with their children. It is also the case that often the alienating parent tells professionals they did not need to go to court, as they and the targeted parent could have sorted things out between them, even though the targeted parent has run out of ways to appease the alienating parent and legal proceedings were a last resort. The parents and children might see many professionals, and the documents might be extensive depending on what allegations have been made and whether Social Services have been involved. In addition, by this stage, it is typically the case that parents are not at their best and are often irritable and agitated.

The situation has led to concerns about the impact of the difficulties on the children who are waiting for the adults involved to bring some resolution for them (1). The harm that is caused by alienating behaviours is difficult to ignore. A court expert will not want to bring further distress to a targeted parent by seeming to validate reports that they have been violent and/or abusive, although all allegations have to be considered and explored. The expert is therefore unable to please both parents and has to try to present the information that they have been given in a way that does not further confuse the situation. In addition, there is hope that experts will offer solutions to what is sometimes an intractable situation. The situation often results in dissatisfaction for all parties involved, including the expert.

DOI: 10.4324/9781003156147-9

The court expert considers all of the information presented to them in the context of the history in the documents and the medical records. The process is as follows:

Letter of instruction

The letter of instruction (LOI) is one of the most important documents sent to the court expert. It outlines the background to the issues and conveys who is involved in the case, what their role is and most importantly, what the court is trying to find out from the assessment. Typically, in the LOI the questions relate to the conflict between the parents, how this is impacting on the children and whether anything can be done to bring about change in their situation.

Background information

The family's situation will be described in the background documents, and each individual involved will have their own account of events. Parents' statements and social workers' and other court professionals' reports are all really important. Medical records are not always available, but if they are, they can be very helpful in producing a more thorough report.

Assessment tools

Experts can use many of the psychometric tests that measure and/or describe IQ, personality, mood, etc., and are already available. Many attempts have been made to try to produce reliable and valid assessment tools for an assessment of PA. It is up to the expert to decide whether to use an assessment tool specifically designed to identify PA or whether they wish to reflect on all the information given and decide themselves whether PA should be referred to. Not everyone accepts the use of the term 'parental alienation', and the difficulties can be described without referring to PA specifically since it is only helpful if it facilitates understanding of behaviours or if it guides clinicians to appropriate interventions.

Measures of parental alienation

The Alienated Family Relationship Scale was piloted to consider the perspective of 493 young adults, who were involved in conflicted family relationships. Seventy-six of the participants were from divorced families, and the other 417 were from intact families (2). The intention was to consider the impact of one parent's open hostility towards another. It was found that the more often young adults perceived alienated relationships within their family, the more distressed and angry they felt towards their parents. Those who felt they had been alienated were also reported to have impairment with attachments and social relationships in general. Young people from divorced families perceived their parents as less able to problem-solve and more likely to alienate each other. It was recognised that the authors of the scale did not have a clinical interview of the participants, which would have been helpful, and the instrument does not appear to have been developed further.

The Relationship Distancing Questionnaire considered the extent to which young people were exposed to parental alienating behaviours (3). They found their instrument was reliable and valid. Sixty-seven percent of their sample came from families who did not have PA as an issue. They acknowledged that the instrument measured the young adult's 'perception' of alienation, rather than whether it actually occurred. Like the Alienated Family Relationship Scale, this instrument has some difficulties in that the data collected was retrospective accounts from young people and so subject to variability in memory, perception, etc.

The Rowlands Parental Alienation Scale attempted to assess the eight areas identified by Gardner by devising a questionnaire for parents to measure the presence and severity of parental alienation in children (4). Of the 592 parents who participated, those who had court findings of parental alienation were more likely to obtain high scores; however, it was recognised that the accuracy of self-reports may be impacted upon by issues like memory, perception, etc., and that this limited the generalisability of the findings. It was felt that the development of a standardised instrument for use during assessment may improve the likelihood of acceptance of PA as a concept and help those evaluating cases in the judicial system.

The Parental Alienation Questionnaire was developed in the hope of producing an instrument that could be used by psychologists assessing PA (5). It was felt that there was a lack of objective measures for psychologists. The eight main criteria originally described by Gardner were used (6), and the psychologists examined the psychometric properties of their scale using descriptions of parental alienation presenting as 'mild, moderate or severe' (7). They found that some of the eight statements were more representative of PA than others. The first of these related to 'unconvincing arguments' not to see the targeted parent, and the second to feelings of 'animosity towards the extended family of the targeted parent', and they referred to this as 'animosity expansion'. They concluded that there were two main factors present in PA and six other factors which were consistent with those highlighted in earlier studies (6). The utility of this instrument remains to be seen. As with all tools there were limitations, and one of the issues related to the use of the instrument with different cultures, as the test was developed in Romania.

Psychometric tests

If the assessment is being carried out by clinical psychologists, they can use valid and reliable instruments to measure other aspects of functioning, for example mood, personality, intellectual ability and/or other measures of cognition if they are believed to be impacting on the parent's presentation.

If there are cognitive issues believed to impact on parenting ability, then these can be assessed, for example memory, planning or aspects of general intellectual ability or social functioning. Measures of parenting ability are typically helpful, as are tests that identify problems with mood. Choosing well-established tests or those considered the 'gold standard' reduces the likelihood of concerns about validity and reliability.

Personality is usually a particularly important aspect of PA, but an assessment of this aspect of functioning is not always requested by the court. Inclusion of this type of assessment is therefore at the discretion of the expert. Personality assessments are often completed and analysed online, and the test developer can produce an online report describing some of the person's personality characteristics. It is, however, up to the assessing clinician to interpret the online report and decide whether to include some aspects of it in their assessment.

Allegations of sexual abuse and other trauma

Allegations of sexual assault and other trauma are common in PA cases and are a source of concern for all professionals involved. This aspect of the assessment is complex, i.e. if the child has been sexually assaulted, they need to be protected and assessed to see whether intervention is likely to be appropriate or helpful for them and if so which intervention is to be recommended. If no abuse has occurred, then the implications of this need to be considered. The same is true for any allegations made by the alienating parent against the targeted parent and relating to physical or emotional abuse of the child or alienating parent.

If the child has not been sexually assaulted but has reported sexual assault to the police, social services, etc., because they want to support the alienating parent, then there has to be some consideration of the impact of this behaviour on them. In some situations, the child will say they have been sexually assaulted, and a forensic assessment is carried out, which at times includes an intimate physical examination of the child. The examination itself can be traumatic and must be considered in the context of other information gathered.

Medical records

Once individuals have given permission for their information to be shared with the legal teams, reviewing the medical records can be very helpful to the court. Parents with a history of personality issues often have an extensive medical file. Personal information does not have to be shared, and the focus is on discussing those aspects of the history that might have led to their current situation and are likely to be helpful in explaining the circumstances, i.e. a history of brain injury, stroke, depression, severe and enduring mental illness, or personality disorder.

Assessment of the family

An assessment involving a combination of interviews, psychometric tests, and review of the court documents and medical records is usually required. The alienating parents are not always happy to give permission for their medical records to be reviewed, although they may make remarks about the targeted parent's medical history. Targeted parents tend to be quite happy for their medical history to be shared. The review is helpful because medical records can contribute to knowledge about the client's history that might be relevant to their assessment. Also, in many cases, the alienating parent attempts to enlist their medical practitioner into supporting their campaign against the targeted parent by describing a list of difficulties that they say the child experiences, or they tell the court the child has a range of problems that prevented them from attending contact, but those are not described in the medical records. Observations of the relationship between the child and their parents may also be required, if the child is agreeable to see the targeted parent.

In my experience it is important to use precisely the same assessment process for both parents, offering them both the same amount of time and psychometric tests to ensure that one parent does not argue the other was offered preferential treatment. The interviews are different because individuals have a history that is unique to them. The parents are likely to make allegations and counter-allegations against each other, and these must be explored. There are circumstances when one parent needs a different type of assessment, for example if they have a neurological condition or have sustained a brain injury likely to impact on cognitive functioning and/or parenting ability, or if a particular issue has been raised, for example someone has complained of memory difficulties, or professionals have noted they are forgetting appointments, etc.

After reading the court documents and the letter of instruction, which outlines which questions are to be answered, the assessor is ready to begin.

The alienating parent's assessment

Parents often present as highly anxious. Alienating parents can also be hostile from the moment they enter the office and may arrive laden with documents that they feel are 'evidence' to support their situation. This is a good time to remind them that the court expert cannot read anything that is not approved by the court. Typically, I start by discussing housekeeping, i.e. breaks, bathrooms, etc., and then setting out the boundaries of confidentiality during the assessment. I also describe what the process will be and how long the assessment is likely to take so that people know what to expect. If psychometric tests are carried out first, it allows a little time to get to know the alienating parent without having any discussion about the emotional factors. The presentation is variable, and people can present as friendly and charming or stern and quiet, with many different combinations of behaviours.

I typically administer the Child Abuse Potential (CAP) Inventory (8), which is a list of 165 questions about parenting and includes measures of reliability as well as a 'lie scale', a 'faking-good' (trying to create a good impression) and a 'faking-bad' (emphasising those aspects of oneself that are unhelpful) scale. There are also measures of consistency and reliability. Unsurprisingly, most parents 'fake-good'. This means their abuse scale is not reliable or valid and cannot be used to indicate the likelihood of abuse. It makes sense that most parents would want to present themselves favourably, but occasionally someone decides to be forthright, and it is helpful to those cases to know that someone is doing their best to engage with the assessment. The psychometric tests can also support the interview, and if the assessor feels that the person is presenting themselves favourably, then it can be helpful to consider the outcome of test scores. If a personality assessment is administered, it is also helpful to consider whether the parent demonstrates 'social desirability' on this measure. Often parents who are 'faking-good' also score highly on social desirability, and some have low disclosure on a personality assessment, which indicates they may not be sharing personal information about themselves. It is good to have this information, and although no single test can be relied upon in court, psychometric tests can be used as supporting evidence and must be considered in the context of an interview and the information in the documents and medical records (if they are available).

A standardised personality test is very helpful as it can provide a lot of information about both adults involved. For example, an individual's personality profile, including their characteristic traits and features, can be derived, and this can help to understand their behaviours. It should be understood in the context of a clinical psychology assessment. There are findings that alienating parents are more likely than others to score highly on a measure of impression management or social desirability, attempt to present as virtuous and have a rigid moral outlook, are overly controlled and try to prevent negative moral judgment (9). Alienating parents have been found to have an unrealistic self-image and be highly sensitive to criticism, even though they deny any negative traits. It has also been reported that they are more extroverted, confident and able to manage social services (9). They did not experience social anxiety and said they were disgusted by violence. Other parents are more flexible and present as less conventional.

Despite saying they abhor violence, during the interview the alienating parent often complains that the targeted parent was violent for many years before they separated from them. This is one of the many contradictions that can baffle unsuspecting experts. They may also offer many recent examples of the behaviour of the targeted parent, even if they have not seen them for many years. In my experience, the alienating parent tends to have difficulty assuming responsibility for their own behaviours and cannot perceive that they are stopping their child from seeing their other parent or that this is a violent act. Sometimes alienating parents deny obstructive behaviours. I have heard many parents tell children, 'I will not love you any less if you see (the targeted parent)'. I then ask them, 'Why would the children think you would love them less if they saw the other parent?' and this does not often gain any response, or the parent says something that does not make sense. The alienating parent might be provocative or churlish and offhand, and it is important for the expert to maintain composure. Sometimes the comments alienating parents make about the expert are very personal. One alienating parent asked me why I remained so 'measured' after numerous attempts to provoke me were unsuccessful. I explained I was remaining objective, and that was why I could not agree with their many negative comments about the targeted parent. They settled down for a short time, before denigrating the targeted parent again.

The alienating parent typically denigrates the targeted parent frequently during the interview. They might accuse them of verbal, physical and/or sexual abuse. They do not like the targeted parent's family and friends, and they say their parenting skills are poor. They say the children do not want to see the targeted parent, and they should be listened to and given a choice. They usually say that if 'everyone left them alone', they might change their minds in the future.

A history of the alienating parent's family situation, academic and occupational experiences, including bullying and mental health, is very important for informing the assessment. Psychometrics are understood in the context of a psychological assessment.

When they are offered professional advice, due to court or Social Services intervention, alienating parents often ignore this, or sometimes they try to use professionals to support their arguments. They do this by misleading professionals, giving information that they believe will support their case. Frequently, this involves suggesting that by permitting the child contact with the absent parent, the young person will be physically harmed. An experienced expert should recognise this, but with the focus on the child's welfare, all professionals are going to be concerned about whether there is some truth in any allegations made, and decision-making about offering advice in these situations can be challenging. In addition, alienators can be charming people who are not always averse to the use of deception to support their position. This highlights the importance of increased awareness of the issues with professionals.

Allegations of violence and abuse, including sexual assault, are observed in many PA cases brought before the courts. There has been a change in thinking about this, as during the 1980s there was concern that allegations of sexual assault made by children had not been appropriately addressed in the past. Therefore, social workers, legal professionals, mental health workers and associated professionals were trained to recognise sexual assault, with a vague premise that 'children do not lie' (10). Although it was recognised that it was important to listen to children, recognise abuse and address the issues, it was subsequently understood that false allegations of sexual assault were made at times, and the impact of this could be significant for the child and the accused. Some studies have reported that a court order to transfer the child to the care of the targeted parent is the only option available when this occurs, assuming the targeted parent has the ability to parent the child (10).

A consideration of whether the alienating parent has had an abnormal grief response or other issue that lends itself to therapeutic intervention can be made. If there are personality issues, these can be described, and the likelihood of interventions being successful can also be reported.

The targeted parent's assessment

In general, the targeted parent presents as more engaged with the process than the alienating parent, and they may arrive with boxes of discovery or lever arch files which have not been approved by the court, and therefore, as mentioned above, they cannot be read by the expert. The targeted parent is typically unobstructive when it is suggested that their medical records should be reviewed. They are usually friendly and engaged with the process, and although there are occasions when they also denigrate the alienating parent and they may be frustrated with the process, these are not their primary concerns. Mostly targeted parents just want to be reunited with their children.

The targeted parent often reports that the alienating parent has prevented them from seeing the children, and sometimes they are bewildered by their experiences. On other occasions, the targeted parent understands their situation and can assume some responsibility for their experiences. At times they show compassion towards the alienating parent, particularly if they remained alone. Sometimes they had contact for years after separating from the alienating parent. On these occasions it is usually the case that the alienating parent met a new partner before contact was discontinued, or the targeted parent met a new partner and the alienating parent then began to understand that they were not going to return to the family. During assessment, the targeted parent may have little knowledge of the child they have not seen recently because often it is years since they had contact with the child. I usually ask the targeted parent for pictures taken before contact stopped, which might reflect the relationship during happier times, and more recently I have also asked the alienating parent to send images, as it can be interesting to see what they consider a 'good' picture to be. These can be very useful, and recently I have noted that when alienating parents send pictures that they perceive to reflect a healthy relationship, I wonder how they selected them, because they are frequently poor and suggest what appears to be a much less satisfactory relationship than the picture sent by the targeted parent.

Often the targeted parent wants advice and is focused on the 'truth', particularly if they have been accused of sexual assault. Sometimes the allegations have been shared with their local schools, social groups and community, so the targeted parent finds themselves in a position of exclusion. They are being punished for something they did not do. It can be particularly difficult for the targeted parent's extended family to cope with this. Many targeted parents cry or become highly distressed when they describe their situation, and less frequently someone becomes angry or frustrated when they express their emotions.

The targeted parent is generally focused on seeing the child and on their welfare. Most targeted parents have suffered emotionally as a result of their experiences. There are occasions when someone wants to see their child but feels the process is too demanding, and I later hear they decided not to pursue the case. This can sometimes be due to financial constraints, although it can also be associated with the demands of another family and relationship, and a parent 'gives up' struggling to try to defend themselves in the face of increasing antagonism.

Assessing the child

Sometimes the alienating parent is so avoidant of professional assessment that they do not bring the child to their assessment. In the past, after one or two non-attendances, I have sometimes managed to arrange to see the child in school if the parent is unable to bring the child to their appointment. Not all schools are agreeable to be involved in any process involving alienation, and sometimes this is because they have been threatened or charmed by the alienating parent.

If the alienating parent brings the child to the assessment, they sometimes arrive distressed and crying or hungry, or very tired and irritable. Assessments in cases where PA is suspected should allow for these eventualities, and the information can be recorded and the appointment re-arranged. Sometimes the alienating parent arrives with other family members who are abusive from the moment they step through the door, even though the child is present and can observe their behaviour. This information can also be described in the report.

A developmental history can be given by the resident (usually alienating) parent. Sometimes this is not consistent with the medical records, but it helps to understand how the alienating parent wishes to present the child at the time of assessment. Sometimes it is said the child never had a good relationship with the targeted parent, who was never interested in them. The medical records may offer a different view and reflect a caring targeted parent who attended many appointments with the child and expressed concerns about them to medical practitioners. It cannot be assumed that someone who presents as a 'caring parent' necessarily behaves that way in private, but professionals are aware of this. Sometimes the medical records indicate that the alienating parent has attempted to draw their doctor into the conflict by asking for diagnoses associated with the targeted parent's behaviour. In one case I was involved with, an alienating parent 'told' the doctor about the targeted parent's poor behaviour and suggested the child had a sore tummy, so they needed to remain home from school the following day, when the court was about to attempt to initiate contact. Not so easily fooled, the doctor asked to see the child alone. When seen alone by the doctor, the child said that they had been told to say they had a sore tummy, but this was not the case. When the alienating parent attempted to say that the child could not attend contact due to a sore tummy, which had required medical intervention, the doctor was able to give an account of their experiences during the appointment, and this was used to inform the court report. There is not always an opportunity for experts to contact the family doctor, but if available, the information provided can be useful.

If the child is old enough, their self-esteem, anxiety levels and mood can all be assessed using a standardised measure, such as the Beck Youth Inventories – Second Edition (11), which measures self-esteem, anxiety, depression, anger and disruptive behaviour. The alienating parent will be keen to attribute any impairment found to the targeted parent's behaviour, even if the child has not seen the targeted parent for many years. The alienating parent does not acknowledge that if a child hears an alienating parent denigrating a targeted parent, this is likely to be stressful for them. Although the alienating parent is likely to deny both this cause and effect, children in protracted proceedings often experience significant emotional dysfunction and rarely experience this issue without some disturbance.

In addition, depending on the history and allegations being made, an assessment of trauma might be required. If the child has been exposed to domestic violence, then they may experience signs and symptoms of an emotional response to a traumatic event. If they have accused a targeted parent of sexual assault but this has not occurred, then when they are asked about their history, in my experience, they usually do not mention the allegations. By the time the child has reached a clinical psychologist, they will have been asked about the allegations by many professionals, and I read the various and sometimes conflicting information given to others and permit the child to choose to report the allegations or not. The assessment is open so the child can say whatever they wish. As far as I remember, no child has ever disclosed sexual abuse to me in a case where PA is suspected, although it has been referred to in the documents on many occasions, and many alienating parents have either alluded to it or said it.

During assessment, I always ask the child to tell me what was the worst thing that ever happened to them. In cases of PA where there have been allegations of sexual assault against a targeted parent, children have often said they had a playground fallout or someone in school bullied them. A meta-analysis of 7893 adults and 1858 children shows that most adults can only discriminate children's lies from the truth at a rate of 54%, although professionals perform slightly better than laypeople (12).

The interview is recorded in detail, and children typically say the targeted parent has behaved badly. They do not want a relationship with them, and they want to be left alone with their alienating parent. They often offer frivolous reasons for not seeing the targeted parent and have few or no positive comments to make about them. For example, one child told me their targeted parent bought them 'a gift card' when he wanted 'vouchers'. I suggested maybe this was really the same thing, and initially the child agreed with me, then, realising they had agreed with me, they immediately changed their mind and said that vouchers were totally different from cards, and this was 'proof' that the targeted parent was not listening to them when they expressed their needs. I suggested to the child that if this was really a stumbling block to contact, I was quite sure the targeted parent would change the card to vouchers. The child said it was 'too late' for changes to be made, and they would have to 'put up' with the card when it was not what they wanted. They would not agree for me to offer the targeted parent the opportunity to change the card.

In the past, I sometimes asked children what their ideal parent would be like. I then suggested that as they had not seen their targeted parent for a long time (before they were old enough to put down long-term memories, in some cases), the targeted individual might have some of the attributes they were looking for in a parent, and perhaps they could meet them and see what they thought. The child often had some preconditions, which usually related to the alienating parent, e.g. buy flowers or chocolates, write a letter of apology, etc., and it was agreed that the targeted parent would do these things and then they would meet. Unfortunately, as soon as the alienating parent understood what was happening, i.e. the child was beginning to relax in relation to their negative thoughts about their situation, they put a stop to any attempt to re-engage the child with their targeted parent, and any expressed wish by the child to meet with them was ignored. I was accused of 'tricking' the child into agreeing to see their targeted parent, even though what had been identified was that the child was willing to give their targeted parent a chance to get to know them if permitted, although only if the alienating parent could be appeased first.

Assessing the relationships

There are usually questions about relationships between the child and their targeted parent. The difficulty is that the child is not usually enjoying a relationship with their targeted parent when they see legal professionals. At best they are 'moderately' alienated, but often cases are in the 'severe' category before they reach court. There is then a quandary about how to observe a relationship that is not being promoted at the time of assessment. If a professional person is not careful, they can become embroiled in trying to persuade the child to see their targeted parent, which, as indicated earlier and consistent with the literature on 'severe' alienation, is typically unsuccessful if they continue to live with the alienating parent. Any unsuccessful attempts to reinstate contact for the purposes of assessment are used by the alienating parent as further proof that the child does not want a relationship with their targeted parent. Attempts can be recorded by the expert, and any obstructive behaviours observed can be noted.

In most cases where supervised contact has been reinstated, much to the alienating parent's disgruntlement, the child tends to be argumentative and difficult, clearly struggling with their role of having to present as not wanting to see the targeted parent, no matter how nicely or kindly the targeted parent presents. In these cases, if there is 'moderate' alienation the child will sometimes begin to engage with the targeted parent, only to present as not wanting to attend contact next time it is due to take place. I have also observed occasions when older children prevent younger children from engaging with the targeted parent and ensure the contact is a negative experience for everyone involved. There have also been cases where an elder child has dragged the younger children away or intervened with any positive contact by shouting abuse at the targeted parent. There are individual differences in the ability of a child to change their behaviour towards the targeted parent and in the relationship that they have with them, and even though two children from the same family might present as having had similar circumstances, they might not always have the same thoughts about reinstating contact. This means that children from the same family could be at different stages of alienation.

Mostly, I have observed cases where arrangements have been made for the targeted parent to see the children, and the alienating parent has intervened to make sure this did not happen. On one occasion it was arranged that two children would see their targeted parent during my assessment, which was to take place over a number of sessions. The alienating parent waited in a car park outside my building and did not know when the targeted parent would join the assessment sessions. The alienating parent did not know I had a side door, and when the children were ready, I asked the targeted parent to join us. The children had previously been averse to seeing the targeted parent, saying he had mistreated them and their alienating parent and would harm them if they saw him. They understood the court was involved in trying to re-establish the relationships, and they had not seen this parent for a number of years, even though he had been their main carer as the other parent had an illness.

When the targeted parent arrived, the children, who were initially reluctant to engage with him, very slowly and carefully began to ask questions about the targeted parent's likes and dislikes and his extended family. The youngest child did not remember the targeted parent at all but was clearly curious and took their lead from the elder child. At the end of the session, I asked the children if they wanted to meet their targeted parent again. The children said they did and even suggested a venue. They gently said goodbye to the targeted parent before I took them back to their alienating parent. Alone with the children, I asked them if they were okay and whether they had any questions or worries. They were smiling and presented as happy and content, although they began to appear anxious as we approached the alienating parent. When I arrived to the car park with the children, the eldest child immediately told the alienating parent that they had seen their targeted parent. The alienating parent walked quickly towards me in a rage, shouting that I had been deceitful in arranging for the children to meet their targeted parent without approval (even though approval had already been given by the court). There was no recognition that the children might be traumatised by the alienating parent's behaviour, and they were exposed to shouting and venomous language as I walked away.

Assessing the relationship between the child and their alienating parent, if it is possible, can be very productive and provide a lot of helpful information. The alienating parent cannot strongly object to this, and obvious reinforcement of negative behaviours towards the targeted parent can be recorded. The alienating parent often makes negative comments about the targeted parent, or if they present as positive towards the targeted parent (which in my experience does not often happen), then the child presents as confused. The child usually knows a lot more about 'court' than they should do, and sometimes they see the professional as an ally of the targeted parent. Once, as one little girl was showing me round her home, she asked if she could run back and ask daddy what she was supposed to tell me again, as she had forgotten. Clearly, the father had prepared her for her conversation with me. Other children have whispered information when I have met them and asked me not to tell the alienating parent what they said. In the presence of the alienating parent, the child has sometimes shouted and complained about the targeted parent and given an entirely different account of their thoughts. This makes for a tough experience when writing the court report, as if the child's views are exposed to the alienating parent, they may be confronted privately.

Unfortunately, some alienating parents are so verbally aggressive and threatening that it is not possible or safe for professionals to observe them with their child. It is interesting to note that although the alienating parent may threaten a professional person, who is an adult and able to walk away, children in the alienating parent's care have no say about the level of dysregulated emotion they are exposed to even if this has been observed by many involved in the case.

Writing the report

Once psychometric tests are scored, the medical records, if available, are reviewed, and the interviews are recorded. It is time to write the report. The reports in cases of PA might be longer than other court reports, and the more information available to the court, the easier it is for them to see how responses to the LOI came about. Interventions can be suggested, and if these are based on evidence, this can be referred to. Even if professionals involved are concerned about the use of the term 'parental alienation', most people agree that some parents interfere with the relationship between a child and their other parent. The point is to try to accurately identify what the issues are, point out any alienating behaviours and propose a relevant and helpful plan for trying to bring about change in the family. It is important to be aware that the evidence showing the likelihood of change for individual therapy in PA is poor. It is also essential to be able to propose possible interventions, and therefore finding a definition of PA that works for everyone is critical. This would enable researchers and clinicians to work together towards finding interventions that protect all parties involved whilst bringing about change.

Self-care for expert witnesses

One of the major issues for professionals is self-care. Alienating parents can be disparaging and threatening, and the work can be exhausting. It can be difficult to continue at times. Sometimes they bring family members to tell the expert what a terrible person they are or gently threaten them, or sometimes they complain about the expert. At times alienating parents ask to speak 'off record', and it is important to refuse this request, although sometimes there are threats, for example, 'if this doesn't work out for me, I'll say you made it all up anyway', which is disheartening. It is important to put these comments into the report so that the assessment is described in full. Often the alienating parent has made similar comments to the other professionals involved in the case, which helps with credibility.

Other experts have had similar experiences in different parts of the world. There are findings that working on PA cases has a significant impact on the welfare of professionals, and they experienced self-doubt, disappointment and anxiety (13). There were occasions when psychologists said that as a result of their experiences, they had decided not to continue with forensic work. It is therefore important for those working on these challenging cases to ensure they look after themselves, have good peer support networks and have appropriate supervision.

Conclusion

The assessment process can be stressful for the children and the parents involved, and it is important for the expert to try to put them at ease quickly, if possible, and explain what format they are likely to be presented with. The limits of confidentiality need to be explained so that everyone involved knows where their information is going to. There should be an expectation of some bumpy times when attempting to assess alienated children, and disparagement of the expert by alienating parents is not unusual. For these reasons good self-care and support networks are important for those working in this complex field.

References

1   Migchels, C. and De Wachter, D. (2017). Parental alienation and the controversy surrounding psychiatric diagnostics. *Tijdschrift Voor Psychiatrie*, 59, 482–488.
2   Laughrea, K. (2002). Alienated family relationship scale: Validation with young adults. *Journal of College Student Psychotherapy*, 17. doi:10.1300/J035v17n01_05.
3   Gerber Moné, J. and Biringen, Z. (2012). Assessing parental alienation: Empirical assessment of college students' recollections of parental alienation during their childhoods. *Journal of Divorce and Remarriage*, 53, 157–177. doi:10.1080/10502556.2012.663265.
4   Rowlands, G.A. (2018). Parental alienation: A measurement tool. *Journal of Divorce and Remarriage*, 60, 316–331. doi:10.1080/10502556.2018.1546031.
5   Sîrbu, A.G., Vintilă, M., Tisu, L., Stefănut, A.M., Tudorel, O.I., Măguran, B. and Toma, R.A. (2021). Parental alienation – development and validation of a behavioural anchor scale. *Sustainability*, 13, 316. doi:10.3390.su13010316.
6   Gardner, R.A. (1998). *The parental alienation syndrome* (2nd edition). Cresskill, NJ: Creative Therapeutics, Inc.
7   Baker, A.J.L. and Chambers, J. (2011). Adult recall of childhood exposure to parental conflict: Unpacking the black box of parental alienation. *Journal of Divorce and Remarriage*, 52, 55–76. doi:10.1080/10502556.2011.534396.
8   Milner, J.S. (1996). *The child abuse (CAP) inventory manual* (2nd edition). New York: Webster.
9   Roma, P., Marchetti, D., Mazza, C., Burla, F. and Verrocchio, M.C. (2020). MMPI profiles of mothers engaged in parental alienation. *Journal of Family Issues*. doi:10.1177/0192513X20918393.
10 Rand, D.C. (1997). The spectrum of parental alienation (Part 1). *American Journal of Forensic Psychology*, 15, 23–52.
11 Beck, J.S., Beck, A.T., Jolly, J.B. and Steer, R.A. (2005). *Beck youth inventories for youth and families manual* (2nd edition). San Antonio, TX: Psychological Corporation.
12 Gongola, J., Scurich, N. and Quas, J.A. (2017). Detecting deception in children: A meta-analysis. *Law and Human Behaviour*, 41, 44–54.
13 Viljoen, M. and Van Rensburg, E. (2014). Exploring the lived experiences of psychologists working with parental alienation syndrome. *Journal of Divorce and Remarriage*, 55, 253–275. doi:10.1080/10502556.2014.901833.

Chapter 10

Existing approaches to intervention

Introduction

Therapeutic 'outcomes' are those aspects of an intervention that bring about positive change. They are typically assessed by collecting data both before and after the intervention has been carried out, analysing it and publishing the results. The results support clinicians with their decision-making about the best therapeutic approach to take when they are attempting to help a family feel more comfortable with their situation. For those who wish to help families in situations involving parental alienation, 'outcomes' are critical. All the research that is carried out is only valuable if it can be used to help understand and improve the experience of families involved in PA. Overall, it seems that no single outcome is appropriate or helpful for all cases, and that is usual for any emotional difficulty or issue. In the case of PA, most professionals involved want to know what can be done to help families in these complex situations and what is likely to achieve the best result for the child involved. In North America some interventions have been developed, and these are described in this chapter. Although they are available in other parts of the world, they are not widely used in the UK.

What combination of interventions are reported to have been effective?

The presentation of alienating parents is often very similar, and the statements made about the targeted parent are markedly alike. The alienating parent is typically highly resistant to change, and although they often say they want the child to have contact with the targeted parent, they might obstruct every single attempt to do this. The presentation suggests that some alienating parents might begin to think that in theory a child having contact with their other parent is a reasonable idea but panic some way through the process as they begin to feel they are losing control. Controlling the situation has been found to be an important part of an alienating parent's repertoire of behaviours (1). Conflict can also happen in a situation where the targeted parent appears triumphant or smug. The situation requires maturity from both parties to achieve success.

DOI: 10.4324/9781003156147-10

In mildly/moderately alienated cases, particularly if the children are young, they can sometimes adjust easily when they see the targeted parent, particularly if they have had a positive relationship with them in the past. If they are taken to contact and are not subjected to the alienating parent's interference, they often slowly relax and engage with the targeted parent. In my clinical experience, a behavioural systematic desensitisation approach can be used to gently increase the amount of exposure the targeted parent has with the child. This approach will also often work with severely alienated children if they are moved to the care of the targeted parent, although it is not always necessary (5). It also depends on the personalities of both the child and targeted parent involved. When children do not remember their targeted parent, they require some time to get to know them, just as they would with anyone they had never met before. Sadly, if the child remains in the care of the alienating parent, then in between contacts, the alienating parent can sometimes undermine the targeted parent and the contact session. This results in professionals having to start again with any introduction process, and it is extremely difficult to try to have a positive contact session when the alienating parent is undermining it.

The older the child is, the more difficult it can be to re-establish relationships, and the more entrenched their beliefs about the targeted parent can be. If adolescents are alienated, they are often on the 'severe' end of the scale, usually because the alienating parent has been able to spend more time with them and they have been subject to more information and stories about the targeted parent's 'poor' behaviour. In addition, they may feel protective towards the alienating parent, particularly if they have indicated the targeted parent is a threat.

To try to understand the cases they saw, a group of social workers considered the information gathered from around 1000 families involved in intractable situations around contact in the courts (2). They felt children were 'brainwashed' into declining an opportunity to engage with their targeted parent and used this language in their writing. They found that therapy was ineffective and sometimes made things worse. Increased time with the targeted parent enabled the child and parent to develop a relationship again, and children reported improvements in other areas of life. Later, when interviewed, the children involved said they were relieved to have been able to reunite with their targeted parent.

Similarly, a follow-up study of 45 children was carried out, in which prior to the evaluation the alienating parent ignored court mandates with impunity (3). The researchers felt the situation was allowed to continue for too long and children needed to be protected from alienating parents. They also found that therapy did not work and caused the relationship to deteriorate. They described a situation when alienation was 'completed', and this meant the alienating parent was the resident parent, the child no longer had contact with the targeted parent but the case remained in court. They noted that to find a therapist supporting the child remaining with their alienating parent was common, and this was based on the premise that separating a child from their preferred (alienating) parent would be harmful to them.

There were also considerations of children who were moved to the care of the targeted parent. It was found that typically at follow-up, they continued to have contact with the alienating parent, unless the alienating parent was too 'disturbed' (it is not clear how this was defined) (3). They found that after removal to the care of the targeted parent, the children were thriving, were engaging better in school and were free to have friendships and enjoy relationships with all of their family members. Children who continued to have contact with the alienating parent sometimes felt burdened and were reported to be more likely to experience emotional disturbance. Changing residence to the care of the targeted parent produced the most efficacious outcome.

Parental alienation reunification programmes (residential)

Reunification centres were developed to help alienated children reunite with their targeted parent. They are spaces where alienated children can engage with evidence-based therapeutic intervention to address any emotional disturbance resulting from their experiences whilst in the care of the alienating parent. Often contact with the alienating parent is stopped to enable the child to recover from any psychological consequence of their experiences. In addition, they can develop a relationship with the targeted parent without interference from the alienating parent. There appear to be a number of similar programmes in the US and Canada and a few in Australia.

Family Bridges workshop

Family Bridges is a four-day workshop that has been running since 1991 to help children reunite with their targeted parents. It is the most well-known workshop and is available widely in the US and Canada. It is also reported to be available in Australia and South Africa (4). It has predominantly been used for severely alienated children, although some moderately and mildly alienated children have also been involved in the programme, particularly since interventions involve the entire family and siblings can present at different stages of alienation. This workshop supports children who have been court-ordered to live with their targeted parent, and the work involved supports them whilst they rebuild their relationships. The child is separated from the alienating parent whilst they build a relationship with the targeted parent. The results associated with attendance at the workshops have been considered and published, and this is one of the few programmes with outcome studies. In a review of 83 severely alienated children, it was found that between 75% and 96% of the children involved overcame their alienation, and their relationship with the targeted parent improved. Beforehand, children had been rejecting their targeted parent for around four to five years (5). In addition to supporting the child with their relationship with the targeted parent, the programme teaches the child and their rejected (targeted) parent to communicate and manage conflict. The child is also taught to remain balanced and be compassionate to both parents, resist outside influence, think critically and be realistic. This programme also appears to be helpful for teenagers who may have thought about their targeted parent negatively for many years beforehand. Over half of the participants in the study were over 14 years old. Interestingly, only a small percentage of the children (4%) changed their view of the aligned (alienating) parent, and it seemed they were able to alter their view of the targeted parent without having to re-align with them to the exclusion of their alienating parent. This is particularly positive given that many alienating parents claim they are concerned about losing the child and appear to feel threatened by the notion that the child will have a relationship with another parent.

Of the small percentage of the children who felt they did not benefit from the programme, complaints were said to have come from those who did not manage to have a successful outcome in reinstating their relationship with their targeted parent, or they became alienated again after the programme ended. All interventions have limitations, and the positive outcomes published suggest that this is one of the most efficacious programmes available.

Overcoming Barriers Family Camp

The Overcoming Barriers Family Camp (6) is a five-day programme that combines psychoeducation and therapeutic intervention in high-conflict families. The programme was developed over several months by forensic psychologists, court personnel, a judge and other legal professionals. Almost all of the ten families who participated were court-ordered to attend against the objection of the alienating parent (6). It seemed that children had not been moved to the care of the targeted parent and remained in the care of the alienating parent. Camp participation was contraindicated by a history of domestic violence, substance misuse, major untreated mental illness and some medical conditions. The families included new partners. They engaged in group-based activities including yoga, cycling, hiking, etc., and although they were in separate groups, both the alienating parent and the targeted parent received psychoeducation as well as some co-parenting sessions to discuss problem-solving issues and develop a future plan. There were group sessions for parents, who discussed their situations.

The children received separate psychoeducation and did some work with the targeted parent to help reunite them. Children were given an opportunity to write down their thoughts about the issues, and targeted parents wrote down their hopes for the future of the relationships. This was followed by some role play. The children bonded with each other and said they felt connected. It was noted that children were never forced to reconnect with a targeted parent. Targeted parents wrote down their thoughts about their children and were able to express how much they loved them. The children read these messages as a group, and without knowing which targeted parent they came from, they described the narratives as 'fake' and generally made negative comments about them. One of the goals for the children was to identify cognitive distortions and recognise how thoughts, feelings and behaviours were related. They also learned how to think about another person's point of view, and there were discussions about trust and safety.

It was noted that with a group of alienating parents, they monitored and commented on each other's behaviour, whereas in the targeted parents group they provided each other with support. At six-month follow-up there were mixed results, and although there was an overall improvement in contact for some families, some targeted parents had either given up trying to have a relationship with their child or had gone back to court. Although the programme was helpful for the families, it did not appear to have necessarily reunited alienated children with their targeted parents, and its utility for severe cases remains uncertain.

Information gathered from 40 parents who had attended the Overcoming Barriers intervention within the previous ten years was considered and examined (7). It was noted that people made positive remarks about the staff, such as 'good therapists who were caring and attentive', noted the 'professionalism of experts' and said, 'the location was lovely', whereas negative comments were said to relate to the setting of the camp, and comments included, 'roughing it is not my thing' (7). Other negative comments related to the cost, and some were disappointed and felt the camp did not offer value for money. There were also concerns from the targeted parent about whether the alienating parent was developing further their alienation skills by learning new methods from other alienating parents. Almost half said the camp did not meet their expectations, and they were disappointed by the lack of follow-up from the court professionals. Overall, the child's contact with both parents increased after attending the camp. The parents were more educated about the impact of strained family relationships, more likely to accept their own contribution to their situation, better able to regulate their emotions, and had improved coping strategies and an improved ability to protect the child from their parental conflicts. Over two-thirds of parents expressed an understanding of the importance for the child of having both parents in their lives. Despite this, over half of those who responded said the level of conflict between the parents remained the same, around one quarter said their relationships had deteriorated and the remainder said they had improved. Therefore, around 25% of respondents said their relationships with their ex-partner deteriorated after attending the camp, and 75% were the same or better (7).

The main difference between the OBFC and Family Bridges is that in the Family Bridges Program the court had ordered the child to be removed to the care of the targeted parent, and there was an effort to ensure a smooth path to reunification, whereas in the OBFC the child remained in the care of the alienating parent.

Family Reflections Reunification Program

A pilot study for the Family Reflections Reunification Program was developed and published (8). It was intended to build on the success of the Family Bridges Workshop and the Overcoming Barriers Program. The programme was designed for situations when traditional therapy had not worked in establishing a relationship between a parent and child aged between eight and 18 years old. It was felt to be unsuitable where estrangement was present due to abuse, neglect, domestic violence, harsh discipline, harm due to a parent's history of drug/alcohol abuse, incarceration or an untreated mental or medical illness of the parent. A group of 12 families with 22 children attended a retreat. Referrals were made by the family court, and there was a court order for suspension of contact between the alienating parent and their child for an undefined 'period of time' until the child was able to resist negative messaging from the alienating parent or until the child's relationship with the non-resident parent improved. Acceptance to the programme also usually required a court order for a change of residence in favour of the non-resident parent, which could be temporary, depending on the alienating parent's response to the intervention. In each case, it had been decided in court that the child should have contact with the targeted parent. The programme ran for four days and five nights.

The FRRP had six processes: (a) the child initially attended the retreat without contact with their parents; (b) the child had psychoeducation; (c) the targeted parent was educated about the programme; (d) the child and targeted parent spent time together, had shared experiences and celebrated their success; (e) the alienating parent had counselling; and (f) a strong continuing care plan was employed, which could include family therapy.

The programme had eight goals, which were to:

1   promote the child's adjustment.
2   improve their critical thinking.
3   help the child understand why alienation happened.
4   help the alienating parent understand how and why alienation happened.
5   work with the family to help develop roles and boundaries.
6   strengthen communication skills between parties involved.
7   maintain the reunification process.
8   continue to promote relationships within the family.

The pilot study was carried out in March 2012. It resulted in a 95% success rate in re-establishing the relationship between the child and targeted parent, usually by the second or third day, and the change in presentation happened quickly. The change was confirmed by the children, parents and observations of the multidisciplinary team. One child, aged 16 years old, did not engage in the retreat and left when one of the parents was diagnosed with a terminal illness. Follow-up took place at three, six, nine and 12-month intervals, and it was found that the children continued to have positive relationships with the targeted parents. This was confirmed by all parties involved and the aftercare team. Findings demonstrated that removing the child from the care of the alienating parent temporarily was not harmful and could be helpful in reuniting the child with the targeted parent. It was noted that the behaviour of the alienating parents had also improved since they attended the programme.

Parental alienation reunification programmes (non-residential)

Sixteen-session group treatment

In a study of 35 participants, the Tel-Aviv Brull Community Mental Health Centre, together with Yale University, developed their own intervention and considered the impact of a 16-session group treatment for PA-associated child anxiety and depression, as well as other issues related to their experiences of parental conflict. The parents in this study were referred by the courts and social welfare authorities, and the targeted parents had not seen their children for at least four months (9). Therapeutic intervention was used to address symptoms of anxiety and depression in the children. Twenty-two out of the 35 children and adolescents referred participated, and there was a partial control group, also of alienated children. Therapy involved cognitive-behavioural therapy, as well as some interpersonal skills training and discussion about coping techniques. Results indicated an improvement in child anxiety and depression at the end of the study, as well as better parental relationships and more cooperation one year after the intervention ended (9).

The Multi-Modal Family Intervention

The Multi-Modal Family Intervention is an intervention based on case management, education, family therapy, individual therapy and coaching (10). All family members are included, and the interventions are aimed at helping modify thinking. A thorough assessment of the child's reasoning for not wishing to engage with the targeted parent is carried out, and an appropriate intervention is chosen. There is an emphasis on understanding the impact of parental separation on the child. In relation to the child, the focus is on modifying black-and-white (all-or-nothing) thinking and developing appropriate coping strategies for periods of emotional distress. In addition, there is some work around changing the family relationships, ensuring that parent/child roles are functional and that co-parenting rules are understood and instigated. A good outcome was one where the child and parent had a relationship that met their capacity to engage with others. It was noted that sometimes therapy proceeded without the alienating parent's engagement or the court's findings or a thorough assessment of whether PA was part of the problem. Despite this there were opportunities for families to bring about change, and it was noted that without the constrictions that might be imposed by other agencies, there was flexibility to proceed and try to find the best outcome for the family involved. The program creators stated these approaches were helpful in increasing the amount of time the child spent with the alienating parent and were also said to reduce alienating behaviours. It was noted that most cases involved hybrid situations (so both parents contributed to the difficulties encountered), and there was an expectation that either enmeshment or estrangement or both existed. It was recognised that a child might naturally align themselves with one particular parent due to having shared interests, gender or temperament, or they might identify more with the parent because they had similar physical or psychological attributes. The parenting style of one parent, if different from another, might also feel more comfortable for the child, or they might have a stronger attachment to one of the parents. During psychotherapy with the preferred (alienating) parent, some consideration was given to whether a parent was needy, dependent or angry or had been traumatised by their experiences, and this was a focus for intervention. Some parents were unaware of the damage there were doing by alienating their children, and education was found to help reduce the frequency of alienating behaviours. This approach also considered whether the child might be enmeshed with their alienating parent, and as a result, the alienating parent would present as a loving parent and the child would appear to be doing very well. Whilst presenting as generally emotionally healthy, the child can also present as clingy and reluctant to be separated and sometimes continues to sleep in the same bed as the alienating parent. An assessment of the child's ability to be separated from the alienated parent then has to be carried out, particularly if some consideration is to be given about moving them to the care of the targeted parent. The risk of moving to the care of a targeted parent is weighed against the damage caused by remaining in an enmeshed relationship. Underlying the enmeshment can be the parent's fear of losing the child, and the parent's neediness is directed towards more appropriate sources than their child. Any issues the child experiences that relate to their feelings of responsibility for the welfare of the alienating parent can be addressed during psychotherapy. The MMFI works towards improving empathy in the alienating parent and reducing frustration and impatience in the targeted parent (10).

Where estrangement occurs as a result of the targeted parent's limitations in respect of sensitivity and emotional regulation, the MMFI can be used to address these issues. It is recognised that targeted parents can present as harsh, controlling and/or immature, and the model attempts to address issues that hinder a resolution. The MMFI model considers whether the targeted parents are compromised to see whether this has contributed to the situation by being unreliable, inattentive and unfocused on the child's needs, or whether a particular personality characteristic is present that causes the child to feel unsafe. If estrangement rather than alienation is present, then the difficulties can be addressed, and the preferred parent can contribute to helping improve the child's relationship with their estranged parent. If the preferred parent is not supportive, then this raises the issue of alienation within the targeted parent/child relationship.

MMFI also claims to be helpful in cases where there is a hybrid situation (11). In these situations, individual psychotherapy is necessary for each individual, as well as careful case management involving a professional likely to be a court representative. The more complex a case is, the more time is needed to try to repair the situation.

Family Restructuring Therapy

Family Restructuring Therapy is intended to be used in high-conflict parental separation (12). It is based on the premise that as all family members are part of the problem, they can also contribute to the solution. The goal is to change the family structure to a shared parenting situation. The focus is on the future, and therapy is action-orientated. It is intended to help families whilst children remain in the care of the preferred parent. There is a book describing the approach, and training is offered (12). Although outcomes of the intervention have not been published, it appears that this programme is likely to be particularly helpful in educating professionals about the difficulties encountered in high-conflict families, including PA. It is reported that there is a significant demand for the programme and that many families find it helpful (12).

Final comments on reunification programmes

All of the above programmes were developed to try to improve the relationships and functioning of the families involved and emphasise the importance of ensuring timely interventions to help those who have experienced the intractable difficulties associated with PA. There have been some negative comments about the workshops, which are sometimes published in the popular press, but it appears that the concerns result from either a misunderstanding of the circumstances surrounding the workshop or a misrepresentation of the programme and associated presentations of some people involved.

From the formal literature it appears that no adult or child is ever forced to participate in the programmes, although the families were court-ordered to attend. Therefore, some might argue that a level of coercion takes place. The programmes have tended to be highly structured with significant professional input, and initially at least, the professionals involved worked pro bono at their camp (6). Family Bridges and Overcoming Barriers rely only on licensed professionals to administer their courses (13). It is noted that licensed professionals adhere to a code of ethics and are aware of appropriate boundaries and standards. They are graduates and have formal training in working with parents and children.

Other family therapy approaches

A family-systems approach has been found to be helpful in mild to moderate cases of alienation (11). The entire family becomes involved in this approach, and various members attend, depending on whether there is a need to focus on particular aspects of the work. There may also be individual sessions, if required, for some family members. It can be difficult for a single therapist to meet the needs of a complex family situation, and therefore a multi-professional approach has been suggested (14). It is also recognised that if the family therapist is required to contribute to any decision-making about when a child should see a targeted parent, this could interfere with engagement (14). For this reason, another individual should be appointed by the court for this purpose. Prior to therapy beginning, a decision should have been made that it is in the child's best interest to have contact with their targeted parent. If the family therapist is seen as an assessor, this can interfere with engagement and can reduce the likelihood of the child and alienating parent speaking openly to them. This is recognised as placing high levels of responsibility on the family therapist, who is expected to aid the child and their targeted parent towards reunification, as well as correct the child's distorted views and improve them, in addition to helping the child in their relationships with both parents (14).

Critical thinking skills

Critical thinking skills are highlighted as an issue by many clinicians interested in rectifying the issues associated with PA. These skills are important for human relationships and problem-solving and reflect the ability to consider a problem, reason and analyse, come to conclusions and be able to problem-solve (15). Critical thinking skills training has been highlighted as an area requiring intervention in alienated children and is included as an important element of many of the programmes described in this chapter. It is felt that it is important for the child to consider and understand why they have been thinking negatively about their targeted parent and extended family. It is also crucial for both parents to understand the process they have been involved in. Experiential camps described in this chapter sometimes teach critical thinking to help the child understand that their targeted parent is not 'all bad', their alienating parent is not 'all good' and all humans have positive and negative aspects of their personality that can be helpful or unhelpful to others. As well as shared activities with the targeted parent, the child receives individual therapy, focusing on education and cognitive restructuring. The aim is to help the child address any cognitive distortions they have associated with the targeted parent. Time with the targeted parent is the optimum way to demonstrate to the child that what they have learned can be reframed or understood another way or that alterations have taken place, and there is an opportunity to bring about change. The child is also supported to communicate their thoughts about their situation, and they may need support to be assertive at this time.

Targeted parents can learn that their child's behaviour is not a reflection of their own thinking but rather they have been manipulated into having beliefs that are not necessarily accurate or true. Alienating parents may be resistant to critical thinking, and it is likely that only in the milder or more moderate cases will they be amenable to any change in thinking. Any change may depend on the reasoning for the alienation. Helping a severely alienating parent to shift their thinking about the child having contact with their targeted parent is likely to be highly challenging.

Spontaneous reunification

Often in severe PA, legal or mental health professionals advise the targeted parent to stop trying to pursue contact, and this advice is often followed, as it is believed to be the least harmful option for the child (14). It is acknowledged that it remains unknown whether the absence of a targeted parent means the child is no longer exposed to denigration and manipulation. It might simply be the case that the child continues to be exposed to a high level of negative expressed emotion and blaming of the targeted parent for any slightly negative event that the alienating parent might encounter.

Also, there are occasions when parents and their children reunite without intervention (14). This sometimes happens when children become more independent from their alienating parent or the parent is no longer in their lives due to serious illness, death or disagreement.

There are findings that when they become adults, alienated children sometimes express a wish that someone had intervened and ensured contact took place in the past (16–17). This has led to the suggestion that if a decision is made not to continue to try to reunite the child with their targeted parent, then an appropriate ending should include a goodbye, and if it is not possible for this to be carried out face-to-face, then a letter should be written by the targeted parent, offering an 'open door' to reunification again at some stage in the future (14). The difficulty with this approach is that some children will refuse to say goodbye to the targeted parent and will not see them to give them this opportunity. Letters can be torn up or thrown away and forgotten about, whilst the alienating parent continues with their denigration and other alienating behaviours.

Conclusion

It is sometimes the case in complex PA presentations that professionals involved prefer to leave the child with the alienating parent, rather than try to address any enmeshed situation or risk any allegations or difficulty associated with separating an apparently high-functioning child from someone who can present as a loving parent. If the child states that they do not want to see the targeted individual and they have their needs met by the alienating parent, it makes it difficult to justify separating them. If they remain in the care of the alienating parent, the child is not required to change residency/school, etc., and this option results in minimum disruption to their lives. The problem with maintaining the status quo is the child is left in the care of an at best misguided and at worst uncaring or emotionally disturbed individual, who is free to model inappropriate behaviour and shape the child's personality without any outside interference.

Practitioners interested in PA point out that it is important to think about how helpless professionals feel when dealing with alienating parents and compare this to the way a child might feel who has no choice but to try to cope with their parent's alienating and other manipulative behaviours (4). The goal of all the therapeutic interventions described is to make the child feel more comfortable and able to manage the situation that they are faced with.

Despite this challenge there is limited access to the specialised programmes that at least understand PA even if they are not always able to bring about change. Education can be an invaluable tool for the entire family, and there is some evidence that it can reduce the frequency of PA behaviours for some children. That is at least a start. It is helpful if alienating parents are given an opportunity to be part of the solution through education and opportunity to change behaviour using therapeutic intervention. Although there is resistance to recognising PA as a form of family abuse, in doing so, there is some progress towards meeting the needs of any child involved in this complex and emotionally demanding family situation.

References

1   Harman, J.J., Maniotes, C.R. and Grubb, C. (2021). Power dynamics in families affected by parental alienation. *Personal Relationships*. doi:10.1111/pere.12392.

2   Clawar, S.S. and Rivlin, B.V. (2013). *Children held hostage: Identifying brainwashed children, presenting a case, and crafting solutions* (2nd edition). Chicago, IL: American Bar Association.

3   Rand, D., Rand, R. and Kopetski, L. (2005). The spectrum of parental alienation syndrome, part III: The Kopetski follow-up study. *The American Journal of Forensic Psychology*, 23, 15–43.

4   Haines, J., Matthewson, M. and Turnbull, M. (2020). *Understanding and managing parental alienation: A guide to assessment and intervention*. Oxon: Routledge.

5   Warshak, R.A. (2019). Reclaiming parent-child relationships: Outcomes of family bridges with alienated children. *Journal of Divorce and Remarriage*, 60, 645–667. doi:10.1080/10502556.2018.1529505.

6   Sullivan, M.J., Ward, P.A. and Deutsch, R. (2010). Overcoming Barriers family camp: A program for high-conflict divorced families where a child is resisting contact with a parent. *Family Court Review*, 48, 116–135. doi:10.1111/j.1744-1617.2009.01293.x.

7   Saini, M. (2019). Strengthening co-parenting relationships to improve strained parent-child relationships: A follow-up study of parents' experiences of attending the Overcoming Barriers program. *Family Court Review*, 57, 224–225.

8   Reay, K.M. (2015). Family reflections: A promising therapeutic program designed to treat severely alienated children and their family system. *The American Journal of Family Therapy*. 43, 197–207. doi:10.1080/01926187.2015.1007769.

9   Toren, P., Bregman, B.L., Zohar-Reich, E., Ben-Amitay, G., Wolmer, L. and Laor, N. (2013). Sixteen-session group treatment for children and adolescents with parental alienation and their parents. *The American Journal of Family Therapy*, 41, 187–197. doi:10.1080/01926187.2012.677651.

10 Johnston, J.R., Walters, M.G. and Friedlander, S. (2001). Therapeutic work with alienated children and their families. *Family Court Review*, 39, 316–333. doi:10.1111/j.174-1617.2001.tb613.x.

11 Friedlander, S. and Walters, M.G. (2010). When a child rejects a parent: Tailoring the intervention to fit the problem. *Family Court Review*, 48, 98–111.

12 Carter, S. (2011). *Family restructuring therapy*. Edmonton, Canada: The High Conflict Institute.

13 Warshak, R.A. (2020). Risks and realities of working with alienated children. *Family Court Review*, 58, 432–455.

14 Fidler, B.J. and Bala, N. (2010). Children resisting post-separation contact with a parent: Concepts, controversies and conundrums. *Family Court Review*, 48, 10–47.

15 Elder, L. and Paul, R. (1994). Critical thinking: Why we must transform our teaching. *Journal of Developmental Education*, 18, 45–35.

16 Baker, A.J.L. (2005). The long-term effects of parental alienation on adult children: A qualitative research study. *The American Journal of Family Therapy*, 33, 289–302.

17 Baker, A.J.L. (2007). *Adult children of parental alienation syndrome: Breaking the ties that bind*. New York: W.W. Norton.

Chapter 11

What other psychological interventions may be helpful in parental alienation?

Introduction

Some authors have referred to parental alienation as a mental health problem (1), and the issues resulting from PA, when it presents at the severe end of the spectrum, are usually associated with emotional challenges and extremely high levels of stress for the family involved. PA is a collection of behaviours that often result from one or both parents' personality characteristics and can have detrimental consequences for the mental health of those who find themselves in this intractable situation. Therefore, it can act as a precipitant to mental illness, in the way any other stressful life event can. Likewise, individuals engaged in PA may have a mental health problem or history which impacts on their behaviour during the process.

Although PA cases are not identical, similar problems arise, and this means recommendations for interventions need to consider the individual presentations. Although the field is in its infancy in terms of understanding approaches to amelioration/treatment, the term 'parental alienation' is beginning to be widely understood and used, and it is therefore important to identify the range of problems that are likely to be observed and note which interventions can be helpful. Generally, interventions for PA have tended to encompass psychoeducation, parenting training for both parents, critical skills teaching for the child, individual therapy for the parents, if required, and group therapeutic intervention, sometimes using cognitive behavioural therapy and/or family therapy (2).

An individual approach for each family member as well as the group is needed. The strength of this approach is that no assumptions are made about the problems that are arising, and the solutions are proposed on an individual basis.

What we know so far

In the largest study of its kind and in an effort to establish 'best practice' for cases involving PA, a systematic review of ten studies written between 1990 and 2015 was carried out (3). There was some reflection on the difficulties encountered by those attempting to study PA. It was noted that there were no clearly defined

DOI: 10.4324/9781003156147-11

outcome measures, there were usually no control groups, the studies were based on non-random samples with retrospective data analyses and these mostly used descriptive statistics. Despite the difficulties associated with comparing studies, the results were interpreted, and the findings were interesting. Most professionals find it difficult to think about separating a child from their preferred parent, and the decision to recommend moving a child to their targeted parent is anxiety-provoking. However, what was established was that removing the child from the care of the alienating parent was not harmful to the child, and it improved relationships with the targeted parent (3). Leaving the child in the care of the alienating parent was unhelpful because it did not lead to a resolution of the difficulties. If the child remained in the care of the alienating parent, they became more severely alienated until the child no longer saw the targeted parent. It was concluded that living with the targeted parent and having limited contact with the alienating parent was better for the child than living with an alienating parent who did not engage with court-ordered intervention.

Professionals making recommendations in cases of PA face a difficult decision-making process and need to assess whether the risk for the child of remaining with the alienating parent outweighs the risk of removal to the targeted parent. If the alienation behaviours are found to be irrational and destructive to the child, then this supports a decision for recommending removal; however, this can be difficult to determine. On the other hand, if the child threatens to self-harm or abscond if they are placed in the care of the targeted parent, this can make it difficult to suggest moving them.

It is therefore important to consider how harmful the situation is to the child and also whether change is likely to bring about an improvement in circumstances or functioning for them, and these issues are the focus of any decision-making in interventions. Studies that describe some of the behavioural aspects of PA have suggested a triage could be helpful, which can begin at the point of assessment (4). This means appropriate interventions can be recommended with suggestions about timescales, numbers of sessions needed and what to do if there is limited or no success in bringing about the change needed.

It is important to recognise that professionals working with PA know that there are ethical issues relating to coercion, and working with PA cases is challenging. Children's rights and civil liberties are very important considerations, and it could be said that court-ordered contact introduces a degree of coercion if the child is not agreeable to attend. Studies that address this issue note it is up to professionals to think about coercion when they make recommendations and refer children to attend contact against their will (5). There is no doubt it is always going to be difficult from an ethical point of view, and although children can sometimes make informed choices, they may not always be aware of the consequences of their actions, which is why children are not allowed to vote, get married, drink alcohol, smoke, drive, etc. Also, they must go to school and attend medical and dental appointments. A decision made by a child not to see their targeted parent must be considered in this context, particularly if it is known that they initially have been manipulated without their knowledge into making decisions that they do not fully understand the consequences of.

In this chapter we will consider how interventions can be used to try to protect children from harm caused by alienation. The overall intention is to improve the child's emotional welfare and meet their needs. Interventions can be used to try to prepare both parents for any changes that are likely to take place. There can be a focus on helping the alienating parent manage their emotions if the child and targeted parent relationship improves. One of the aims of the intervention can be to develop or repair the co-parenting relationship if this is possible. Ultimately, professionals want to improve the situation for the child, whilst at the same time try to ameliorate any distress experienced by any party involved.

Families involved in mild parental alienation are less likely to be seen in court than moderate or severe cases. In these cases, the alienating parent may be una-ware of any harm they are causing and be simply fed up with the targeted parent. Psychoeducation can be helpful at this stage to help the family understand the pro-cess that they are involved in. Moderate and severe PA is likely to require a higher level of intervention, such as removal from the preferred parent. The interventions proposed are suggestions for situations involving PA and might be utilised instead of, alongside or after removal, if this is indicated.

If the child is removed from the care of the alienating parent, then transfer to a transitional home, e.g. grandparents, extended family/friend or, in some cases, foster care, is sometimes indicated for some children involved in complex cases. Once the child has reunited with the targeted parent, then the alienating parent can be gradually re-introduced with initially supervised access to ensure alienation does not occur again. Those who are supervising alienating parents would have to be educated about PA and make a commitment to report any concerns about behaviours during the contact period.

Typical problems requiring intervention for the alienating parent

The alienating parent sometimes behaves in a way that makes it difficult for pro-fessionals to show compassion for them, particularly if they believe the profes-sional is 'not on their side', as they see it. Therefore, they vent their anger towards the professional (5). It is understood by most working with PA cases that typically the alienating parent presents with emotional or personality disturbance. They might have made either malicious or strongly believed allegations against the targeted parent that, despite repeated investigations, have not been substantiated. Whether a credible risk exists will have been thoroughly and appropriately con-sidered, although some alienating parents say they do not believe the outcomes if their accusations are not supported.

The alienating parent will often experience one or more of the following:

- Resistance to change
- Problems with adjustment/grief and loss

- Fear of being alone and high dependency needs
- Other personality issues and a lack of empathy for others
- Feelings of revenge/anger with the targeted parent for leaving them
- A struggle to assume responsibility for their part in the situation
- A lack of knowledge about or seeming not to understand the impact of events on their child

Typical problems requiring intervention for the child

Some children present as frightened of their targeted parent in PA, and fear could be an area for consideration in interventions, particularly if the alienating parent has decided to engage with the process of change and is prepared to model a lack of fear with the targeted parent. Other present as angry and refuse to discuss the issue or even sometimes to use the targeted parent's name.

In PA the child can experience one or more of the following:

- A level of paranoia relating to the targeted parent's motives and intentions
- Anger when the targeted parent's name is mentioned, or other symptoms more often associated with exposure to trauma
- Adjustment issues associated with the parents' separation/conflict
- Emotional difficulties associated with exposure to conflict
- Difficulty expressing empathy for the targeted parent
- Problems critically analysing their situation

Some of the decision-making around intervention for the child might be associated with whether any shift in behaviour or thinking was observed in the alienating parent.

Typical problems requiring intervention for the targeted parent

Some thought will always have been given by professionals as to whether there is an element of estrangement and/or whether the targeted parent has contributed to their situation through frustrated and angry behaviours or verbal exchanges (known as a hybrid situation). Also, the targeted parent can at times have higher expectations of the child than are reasonable.

The targeted parent will often experience one or more of the following:

- Grief and loss associated with the struggle involved
- Frustration with the situation and with the alienating parent and child
- Stress associated with their experiences

In hybrid cases the targeted parent might have contributed to their situation by speaking aggressively or behaving poorly towards the alienating parent, particularly if they have become frustrated with the process, in which case the following must be considered:

- Dealing with emotional dysregulation
- Education about the impact of events on the child
- Ability to express empathy for the alienating parent
- Difficulty assuming responsibility for their contribution to the relationship ending

The issues described can be discussed within psychoeducation and each difficulty addressed.

Documents and information for the therapist

There must be agreement beforehand about what therapeutic approach/intervention is required and what the goals are, which documents are to be shared and with whom. Any assessment of the family members that recommends intervention/therapy should be forwarded to the professional involved, so that they can understand the expert's perspective. This will usually include background on the client, so the professional does not have to spend as much time gathering this information as they would usually, although they may wish to qualify some of the detail. When the professional is approached there should be a clear outline of what is required, with some flexibility in case events have changed since the assessment was conducted.

Psychoeducation for parents

Education can be carried out individually, or the parents can be seen together. In severe alienation, this might not be possible due to either or both parents' problems with emotional dysregulation and conflict. Psychoeducation for parental alienation begins by describing the boundaries for those involved and the process of the intervention. The alienating parent might not be aware of their responsibilities as a parent, and this can be outlined for them. Adjustment will have been required by all parties involved, and this can be recognised as a commonality within the PA framework.

Some education about the impact of parental conflict on the child is a good place to begin. There also needs to be some discussion about the implications for the child if they do not have contact with the targeted parent. This needs to be delivered in a way that does not make the alienating parent feel judged or that their role is diminished. The child needs both their parents, and the alienating parent can benefit from the child's engagement with the targeted parent. They are likely to have a happier child if they are no longer exposed to parental conflict, and both parents involved will have more time to consider other activities if parenting is shared.

The likelihood of the child changing the way they feel about the alienating parent, if they are supported to see their targeted parent, needs to be addressed so that the alienating parent can feel reassured and supported that their child will not love them less if they see their other parent.

Parents who engage in moderate or severe alienating behaviours are often in a high state of alert and sometimes use the word 'threat' when referring to the targeted parent. Reassurance tends to be unhelpful. Alienating parents can find it alarming if their children exhibit features of the other parent or their extended family and try to quash them. These features can result from a genetic propensity to present in a similar fashion to the targeted parent. Some alienating parents hope to reduce the likelihood of the targeted parent's features developing by restricting access to the other parent. Education is important because alienating parents can be helped to understand that there are likely to be genetic traits of the other parent evident no matter what they do, and by trying to inhibit these, they are more likely to harm the child than help them. If they denigrate the targeted parent, personality traits that do not 'fit' comfortably with the alienating parent might be exhibited by the child, which is likely to be stressful for them. The expression 'you're just like . . .', with negative connotations, is likely to be hurtful to the child, and continued critical comments can impact on self-esteem.

Some parents fail to demonstrate empathy and cannot always be helped to see their child's point of view. This is likely to be identified during their assessment. If an alienating parent does not demonstrate the ability to have empathy with their child or a targeted parent, then this can be addressed. Education about the impact on the child of modelling a lack of empathy towards others is essential. Issues associated with modelling and practicing empathy can be discussed, as this is a significant issue in PA. Typically, empathy has been found to be a learned quality (6–7), and it is essential for many aspects of morality and social interactions, including prosocial behaviour. Cognitive empathy in particular (the ability to understand the emotions of others) has been found to be influenced mostly by environmental factors and is helpful in all social exchanges (8). Therefore, this is an important aspect of functioning for the development of the child, and the alienating parent needs to be able to demonstrate to the child that they have empathy for the targeted parent and understand that rejection is likely to be hurtful for them.

Like the alienating parent, the targeted parent is required to cope with a lot of information about their responsibilities and the needs of the child. The individual delivering the education has to be sensitive to any discomfort the targeted parent might feel relating to periods when they did not pursue contact or felt unable to try to reach out to their child. It is usually the case that targeted parents go through periods when they are frustrated with the process or do not know how to proceed. During that time, they might think about their child but are unable to contact them and often feel powerless to bring about change. The targeted parent might also worry about others' perception of them, relating to their own feelings of whether they 'tried hard enough'. Also, the targeted parent must be able to manage any feelings of resentment towards the alienating parent and/or their child and understand that these feelings are 'normal' for many people.

It is important to consider the goals of the intervention, so that both parents can begin to think about the projected outcome if they engage or do not. Some discussion can be had about how the family might present after the intervention has been completed and what their various roles might be. Alienating parents involved in this situation might base their decisions about the future care of their child on their past experiences with the targeted parent. It could be argued that is all they have at this stage, but there should be some consideration about the possibility that individuals involved have changed their views on some aspects of parenting, and this can be discussed. Individuals can offer their thoughts about how the situation might proceed or make suggestions about the outcome. If severe alienation is present, then this might be difficult, and there might not be any agreement about the future outcome, or the alienating parent might not engage in any joint education sessions.

Comprehensive parenting classes are widely available and can also be very useful in helping those involved understand (a) their responsibilities and (b) the appropriate role of a parent.

Psychoeducation specifically for children

Within the court system, the wishes and feelings of the child are considered, and the child's welfare is paramount. The child will typically say they do not want to see the targeted parent, and practitioners will try to bring about change and repair the relationship, although this is not straightforward.

Some authors have suggested that in dealing with complex cases, if a child is asked directly whether they have a story to tell, the therapist may gain some awareness of the narrative (story) that they have been asked to repeat (if this has occurred) (9). Most children involved in PA have a story, which they can only vaguely explain but which typically includes comments such as, 'they were bad to my (other parent)', or 'they hit me' or 'broke my toys', etc. Without sight of the court documents these comments would raise concerns with professionals about whether they are supporting a child to reunite with an abusive parent. It is therefore important for the professional involved to be informed about the background.

In relation to psychoeducation for children, they can find it helpful to hear that their parents once loved/liked each other (if they did). Children tend to understand that not all parents remain in a relationship together and that often when they separate it is because they have irreconcilable differences, and this does not necessarily mean that the child cannot have a relationship with both parents or that they love them any less. They also tend to know that when people 'fall out' they typically say things about each other that they would not usually say. They see this often in the playground, and this is part of everyday life. The child's emotional journey can be normalised, and they can be offered information about the experiences of other young people so they know that their feelings are not unusual and do not reflect poor ability to cope with events in their lives.

If the child remains in the care of the alienating parent whilst intervention is carried out, then that parent will bring them to sessions. They usually will not agree to anyone else getting involved. The alienating parent tends to change the appointments frequently or does not attend at times. In this way they retain control of the child, who at this stage is unlikely to see their targeted parent (although it varies from case to case). It is therefore important for professionals to be prepared for cancellations at short notice or for the alienating parent to say that they had turned up but the professional was not available, even if they were sitting looking out the window whilst waiting for the alienating parent and child to arrive.

Typically, in PA, children are not able to demonstrate the ability to see the targeted parent's point of view or have empathy for them. If they are asked to list the problems with their targeted parent and how they would like that parent to be, they often say they do not know (some hesitate and appear suspicious). They can then be asked to think about another parent that they like, perhaps a parent of someone at school, and describe the attributes that they find attractive in that parent. Then they can be asked for a list of all the things they like about their 'favourite' (alienating) parent. When asked, they often say they wish their targeted parent could be more like their alienating parent. This is important information for intervention, as it describes those attributes that the child values and can be a platform from which to explore and think about personality qualities present in both the child and their parents.

Often children say their targeted parent cannot do anything to repair the situation, although sometimes they ask the targeted parent to apologise to the alienating parent. This does not mean they will change their view, but it demonstrates to the child that the targeted parent is willing to work with them. The targeted parent is usually happy to comply. If the alienating parent remains opposed to the reunification, they will typically interfere with any attempts to smooth things over.

Critical thinking skills

Critical thinking skills involve the ability to make expert judgements. Involving the ability to analyse information and form conclusions, they are highly relevant and important in education and essential in everyday life. It is believed they can be learned or improved by most people (10). Critical thinking skills can be used in PA if those involved have all the information they need to form opinions and provided there is no interference from outside influences, such as an alienating parent. These skills can be a particularly helpful development in PA, since they support the child to think about their situation, look at balanced evidence from a range of sources and form conclusions. The intention is to help them see that no parent is 'all bad' or 'all good'. Critical thinking skills are typically taught after the child has been removed from the alienating parent (5).

In addition, it is noted that there is no perfect parent/child relationship, and each will have good and bad qualities (4). It is important to be able to recognise, accept and integrate these factors, and depending on the age of the child, this can be an area for discussion.

Confidentiality in court-instructed interventions/therapies

The confidentiality in a court assessment is different to the levels employed in other situations, as the information can be shared with the court. In court-ordered therapy/intervention the court needs to be advised about the progress or otherwise. However, the client needs to know their information is not being widely shared; otherwise there may be difficulties with engagement. For this reason, it is usually helpful to explain to the client at the outset that the level of progress will be shared with the court but that the information discussed in the session will not. The client feels safer talking about their personal information without worrying about whether their ex-partner or others will know the details of their sessions.

Motivational interviewing

Motivational interviewing (MI) is a form of counselling that can be used to initiate a person's own motivation to change and adhere to intervention (11). It is often used for those cases who are resistant to change and wish to take control themselves, like most alienating parents in PA. MI can help an alienating parent consider and reflect on change. In these circumstances, it can be used to help the alienating parent understand the reasons for their behaviours. It is based on listening to the person's reasons for resisting change, then using empathy and guidance to help them shift towards a more productive situation, rather than telling them what to do. It also offers an opportunity for people to vent, think about their situation and describe how they feel in a confidential setting.

MI can be a good starting point for PA as it helps the therapist understand the client and the reasons for their behaviour. MI alone is unlikely to bring about sufficient change in PA, but it can help with engagement.

Grief, loss and adjustment

Many parents involved in PA are struggling to adjust to the loss of their partner and also change in their expectations for the future. Psychological interventions are helpful in addressing issues relating to grief, loss and adjustment and can be instigated with each parent in individual therapy (12). The professional person involved can reflect on the issues facing the family members and see whether this type of approach might work best for them. Most therapists can incorporate an element of helping the parents to adjust to their new circumstances, no matter what their preferred therapeutic background is.

Cognitive behavioural therapy

Cognitive behavioural therapy (CBT) is a highly structured and pragmatic therapeutic approach that involves working with the client in a collaborative way to identify troubling thoughts and challenge negative assumptions. It involves look-ing at how behaviours, thoughts and feelings are connected and understanding how negative cycles can be stopped.

CBT was initially found to be successful with anxiety and depression and was developed for a number of other emotional difficulties including phobias, panic disorder, post-traumatic stress disorder, eating disorders, sleep problems and the management of chronic pain (13–14). In PA it could be used to help both the adults and the children who experience emotional difficulties resulting from their experiences or struggle to manage the associated conflict.

Family therapy

Family therapy is a type of counselling that involves family members attempting to improve relationships, address conflict and create a functional situation. There is evidence for its use in complex family problems (15–16). Since the issues in families often relate to structure, roles and boundaries, it has been considered a helpful approach in PA. It has been argued that family therapy in its traditional form is not helpful to PA and can be harmful at times (5). Therefore, a modified form has emerged and is used by many involved in PA work (3).

In cases of PA, modified family therapy usually involves all the members including step-parents, step-children, etc. Modified family therapy remains a valid and highly valued approach for conflictual families; however, it seems that the issues associated with the difficulties that PA presents with are not being met for all cases by this approach. Many severely alienated families attempt family therapy on several occasions and do not progress, and therefore a new approach to intractable cases is required.

Using third-wave psychological therapies for parental alienation

The list below is not exhaustive, and therapies described do not represent all the new third wave of interventions available. Therefore, there may be other approaches not described here that would be helpful with a particular problem in PA that might be relatively unique to one individual.

Dialectical behavioural therapy

Dialectical behavioural therapy (DBT) was developed to help people who were at high risk of self-harm or suicide and were difficult to treat (17). It has been found to be particularly helpful with people who have personality difficulties, including those who have trouble regulating their emotions. It involves group and individual therapy and enables people to focus on the core skills of mindfulness, distress tolerance (helping the person understand themselves and their situation), interpersonal effectiveness (respecting the self whilst communicating with others) and emotional regulation.

DBT has the potential to be particularly helpful with the alienating parent in PA, who often has difficulty regulating their emotions and can struggle to manage feelings of distress experienced when they are separated from their child or to communicate effectively with the targeted parent and/or their child. It could also be helpful in hybrid cases where the targeted parent struggles with emotional regulation. Mindfulness can be used to help soothe emotional distress associated with separation for either parent from the child.

In relation to high-dependency needs, alienating parents who have these difficulties can focus on this, and they can be helped to understand the source of their difficulties and what they can do to self-soothe. For parents who are narcissistic, this approach is also going to be helpful, particularly when addressing issues with empathy and self-focus.

Compassion-focused therapy

Compassion-focused therapy (CFT) emphasises the need for 'self-compassion' as well as having compassion for others and being sensitive to receiving compassion from others (18). CFT was developed to help those who struggle with shame and self-criticism and who come from backgrounds of negativity. Mindfulness also plays an important role when this therapeutic approach is used.

Although many alienators come from backgrounds of negativity or might have been alienated themselves, they often struggle to recognise any harm that they have experienced as a result. This is particularly the case if they are enmeshed (highly involved) with their own parents. Typically, alienating parents do not say that their parents/carers have failed to protect them. However, some people who have grown up in harsh or critical environments have not developed the ability to self-soothe in a way that is easily accessible to them.

CFT s a method whereby engaging with painful memories and working with the fear of compassion from others can be a focus of therapeutic intervention. Also, by learning to accept compassion and have compassion, we can become compassionate towards ourselves. Sometimes when CBT does not work, it is because people are so used to being condemned that they cannot accept that a change of thoughts can be kind and give the person permission to 'feel' positive emotions. CFT developed from CBT, with a focus on using kind inner thoughts when tackling negative automatic thoughts.

CFT recognises the relevance of attention, reasoning and rumination, behaviour, emotions, motives and imagery. The goal of the therapist is to help the client to feel together and connected with them, so like CBT, it is a collaboration.

Whilst CFT is a shared experience for the client and therapist, it is important for the therapist to remain in control of the sessions, and this can be particularly difficult with PA cases where the alienators are frequently used to asserting themselves. Clients like this are sometimes frightened of their own ability to push people away from them (18). Therapists need to set boundaries, be honest and give clients what they need rather than what they want. For this reason, support is highly important for therapists working with this client group.

The client group, who in this case are likely to be those who alienate their children from others, may have a fundamental belief that others are 'blaming' them for their situation, and whilst they 'blame' others, they may actually believe deep down that their situation is their 'fault', i.e. 'if I hadn't shown them my real self, they wouldn't have left me'. For these individuals, sometimes they view kindness as an indulgence. The function of CFT is to help people stand back from their feelings and give themselves more compassion, and in a sense, it involves relearning how to think.

CFT is relevant in alienation, because those who alienate children are typically resistant to permitting others to help them. They state that everything would be okay if everyone would 'go away and leave them alone', even though when this happens, it is often the case that the alienating parent struggles with children who have been damaged by the parent's behaviours and associated exposure to conflict.

Although there is no research evidence for the efficacy of CFT in alienating parents in PA, treating parents in this way offers them the opportunity to accept compassion and learn how to be compassionate towards their children.

The goal in all of this is to teach the alienating parent to have compassion for themselves and for their children, so that they can provide the optimum parenting experience for the children and permit their children to have a relationship with a (usually) previously loved targeted parent, rather than damage the child by using them to hurt an ex-partner.

CFT helps people consider whether they use one feeling, such as anger, to block out other emotions associated with threat, i.e. powerlessness, grief, loss and/or sadness. It is easy to see how this could be relevant for those who have recently had a partner decide to leave them. Humans typically want to feel safe and cared for, and it is reported this is central to CFT because of the association with feelings of wellness. It is referred to as a 'soothing and contentment' system (18).

Feeling safe is therefore a goal in this therapy, and it is described as contentment and being 'at peace with oneself', which some people seek by isolation or keeping their distance from others. This is believed to be because some people are frightened and resistant to receiving care and being soothed by others.

What is interesting about CFT for this client group is it focuses on considering the individual's threat, levels of excitement and soothing systems, rather than blaming them (which they may have had a lot of, particularly if they have been involved in proceedings for a while). Therapy works towards helping the individuals involved address their issues in a compassionate way by explaining that the brain is complex, and their presentation can be explained by a combination of genetic dispositions and emotional memories from their social worlds. So they are being helped to address an issue for which they are not responsible and to show compassion for others, including their children. In doing this, people are asked to take responsibility for cultivating and changing their thoughts to enable them to function better. The idea is that over time, people take more responsibility for change and view setbacks for what they are but do not allow them to become an indicator of the likely outcome.

In CFT, the parent is encouraged to disengage with threat stimulations, e.g. self-criticism and anger, and focus instead on compassion, mindfully standing back from waves of emotion and changing to gentler refocus and imagery. They can then engage with adverse or avoided memories through a kinder lens.

Shame is associated with threat, and this is something that can be worked with in PA. One issue which is not always congruent with PA is the importance of guilt in CFT. In CFT guilt should be considered and tolerated, whereas in PA it is not an emotion experienced by everyone who alienates their children.

It is believed that through the use of CFT, the client can reduce threat by accepting feelings for what they are, having self-compassion and self-understanding, recognising negative self-criticism and refocusing away from this, and finally recognising rumination that is unhelpful and replacing it with positive compassion focus and practice (18).

It should be recognised that CFT has not yet been proven as an evidence-based therapeutic intervention; however, the few small studies that have been carried out have had positive outcomes (19–20). This is encouraging particularly as CFT shows promise in the treatment of low self-esteem (21), which is an issue for some people involved in PA (22).

Acceptance and commitment therapy

Acceptance and commitment therapy (ACT) is based on behavioural therapy and was initially created by Hayes in the mid-80s and further developed by Wilson and Strosahl (23). It involves taking 'mindful' action and being the person you want to be. The aim is to improve wellbeing and functioning, and it involves improving quality of life whilst managing the pain that accompanies the everyday. The core principles of this approach are mindfulness (living in the present moment), defusion (separating from thoughts, images and memories), acceptance of unwanted experiences, noticing the self as a person who is aware and thinks, values (thinking about how the person wants to represent themselves) and committed action (living by those values). ACT has been found to be efficacious in a wide range of psychological problems including psychological flexibility (ability to cope with change) (24), and there is also evidence for its use when supporting parents who are dealing with a wide range of child-related issues (25). Both of these aspects of functioning are particularly important in PA.

ACT can be helpful in PA when attempting to support both parents to cope with the stress associated with their situation. Within a therapeutic environment, individuals involved can consider whether they have contributed to the event, how they wish to continue and what the likely outcome will be if they engage with change.

Mindfulness

Mindfulness is a way of managing stress and involves being fully present in the moment and not allowing distracting thoughts to interfere with how we feel. Judgements are noted and allowed to dissipate. Mindfulness can be used within therapy or as an accessible intervention for anyone who wants to address stressful life events. It improves wellbeing, reduces emotional reactivity and improves behavioural regulation (26). It can be particularly helpful in addressing feelings of anxiety and is therefore likely to be helpful for those experiencing stress associated with PA. It is likely to be helpful for all parties involved, including professionals.

In relation to revenge, research has shown that forgiveness has been found to offer the most favourable outcome for those who feel they have been wronged (27). Mindfulness meditation has been found to be helpful in reducing anger rumination and leading to greater forgiveness (28). It is therefore likely to be particularly helpful for any parent who feels they have been wronged in the process involved in PA.

Behavioural add-ons

Behavioural therapy is based on learning theory, which utilises what is known about how behaviours develop and uses this information to bring about behavioural change. From a behavioural point of view, it is likely to be helpful if the alienating parent pairs a positive event, e.g. yoga or attendance at another sporting or social event, with the child going to the targeted parent, so that as well as being soothed they are rewarded. The targeted parent and child could bring the alienating parent back something to show the child has not forgotten them, like a shell from the beach or a special leaf or flower from a walk. This has the benefit of teaching the child to be thoughtful about others, and although the situation results from the parent's struggle, it is important to try to remain focused on what the child is learning from their experiences.

What combination of events can be considered?

In severely alienated families, the alienating parent is highly resistant to change, and even when they say they want the child to have contact with the targeted parent, they often obstruct every single attempt to support contact. The older the child is, the more difficult it can be to re-establish relationships. Younger children can be taken to contact and are often flexible in their approach to relationships, so that they will work with what has been presented to them, i.e. if someone treats them nicely, they will respond positively.

It has been suggested that another option, which would not involve a permanent move of home for the child, could occur if the child spent an extended period of time with the targeted parent, so that they could build their relationship again (4).

This could take place over a holiday period, for example during the summer months, and the child then returns to the care of the alienating parent afterwards. This allows the targeted parent and child time to enjoy rebuilding their relationship without any interruptions from the alienating parent. Unfortunately, there is a possibility that the alienating parent will begin to manipulate the child again when they return to their care. As a result, the child might begin to reject the targeted parent again, and with severely alienating cases this seems unlikely to be successful. It may work with moderately alienated children.

Another option that I have seen work very well for some families is when the child is removed to the care of the targeted family or their extended family, whilst the alienating parent completes some intervention with the intention of returning to a shared-care arrangement with both parents once the work has been completed. This gives the alienating parent the opportunity to have the child returned to their care. The alienating parent (and sometimes their extended family and/or partner) continues to have supervised contact with the child whilst they complete the work, and although they are not living together, the child has stability in that they continue to see their alienating parent and can develop their relationship with the targeted parent and their extended family without interference. When work has been completed satisfactorily, the alienating parent and targeted parent can gradually return to a shared-care arrangement. This approach requires the support of professionals since the child needs to be able to communicate any concerns about their situation as it changes.

Table 11.1 Psychological Therapy Approaches in Parental Alienation

Alienating Parent Issues	Intervention
Resistance to change	Motivational Interviewing CFT
Adjustment, grief and loss, anger, revenge	Grief counselling or ACT for grief and loss
Personality, i.e. lack of empathy, high dependency needs, blaming others	DBT or modified CBT
Parenting	Parenting education
Coping ability	Mindfulness/ACT/CFT
Child Issues	
Critical skills thinking, i.e. induction of paranoia, lack of empathy, etc.	Psychoeducation
Emotional disturbance/adjustment	CBT
Coping ability	Mindfulness
Targeted Parent Issues	
Adjustment, grief and loss, anger, revenge	Counselling or ACT for grief and loss
Personality, i.e. blaming others, emotional regulation	Modified CBT or DBT
Parenting	Parenting education
Coping ability	Mindfulness, ACT or CFT

If all else fails

In some severe cases, where there is no opportunity to try to bring about change and a decision is made that the child is going to remain in the care of the alienating parent, then the targeted parent can have a planned goodbye.

This gives the targeted parent an opportunity to tell the child that they love them and that they can be contacted in the future. They can agree on whether the targeted parent is to send cards/gifts for birthdays and other holidays. The child may reject all these offers, but if the targeted parent has suggested that they will continue to support and care for them, then the child is less likely to feel that the targeted parent has simply disappeared.

If there is no opportunity for the targeted parent to speak to the child, then they may be offered an opportunity to craft a 'goodbye for now' letter, advising that they can be contacted in the future if the child wants to see them and outlining what arrangements have been made for birthdays, holiday cards and gifts so that the child knows what the arrangement is and does not feel that they have been forgotten about. The letter will need to be read to the child by another professional and not an alienating parent.

If the child is too young to participate in or remember this event, then other arrangements need to be made. For example, the child's solicitor or social worker (if there is one) would need to agree to accept a letter from the targeted parent and read it to the child once a year, for example around the time of their birthday. The letter can include age-appropriate information about the targeted parent, so the child knows what their other family is doing. Episodic memory (memory for events containing information such as 'when', 'what' and 'where') begins to mature at around age six and has completed in typically developing children by around nine years of age (29). If the child is typically developing, then after their ninth birthday they should no longer need to be reminded every year that their targeted parent wants contact with them, as they should remember the annual meetings. If they are nine years old or older at the time of the event, then at least one reading should be provided for them. It would seem prudent for the professional reading the letter to ask the child whether they would like the arrangement to continue. This reduces the likelihood of the child feeling abandoned and should provide some confirmation to them about their targeted parent's commitment. They will know that they have been loved.

The alienating parent might object to the reading of any correspondence from the targeted parent and may re-interpret the letter later when alone with the child. As this is most likely to take place in severely alienated cases, it is probably best if the child does not take the letter away with them unless they feel very strongly that they want it. This approach offers the child an opportunity to have their own interpretation of the correspondence, and by reading it every year until they are at least nine years old (in a child with typical development), then at least they will remember that the targeted parent attempted to remain in contact with them.

There should be an arrangement for school reports, pictures, etc., to be forwarded to the targeted parent and for any significant medical events to be reported, for example hospital attendance. What determines a significant event will need to be decided beforehand.

Conclusion

Modified family therapy has been the approach to intervention in PA for many years. Studies show it has been helpful in mild and moderate cases, although not for severe alienation when the child remains in the care of the alienating parent. Modified family therapy continues to be utilised in these mild to moderate cases with some success, depending on the severity of the cases and whether the child has been moved to the care of the targeted parent.

The issues are significant and cause high levels of distress for individuals involved, and attempts to try to use other evidence-based interventions have not yet been fully considered. With an awareness of the issues and a focus on evidence-based practice, cases can be approached individually using appropriate interventions. This is likely to be helpful in leading to the shift needed in current practice and in supporting the many parents who struggle to manage this intractable situation.

This chapter is an attempt to suggest mainstream therapeutic intervention for the more complex, intractable family cases. It involves using proven therapeutic interventions in problems experienced by those who are immersed in PA.

References

1 Lorandos, D. and Bernet, W. (2020). *Parental alienation: Science and law*. Springfield, IL: Charles C. Thomas Publisher.
2 Warshak, R.A. (2020). Risk and realities of working with alienated children. *Family Court Review*, 58, 432–455.
3 Templer, K., Matthewson, M., Haines, J. and Cox, G. (2016). Recommendations for best practice in response to parental alienation: Findings from a systematic review. *Journal of Family Therapy*, 39, 103–122. doi:10.1111/1467-6427.12137.
4 Fidler, B.J. and Bala, N. (2010). Children resisting postseparation contact with a parent: Concepts, controversies and conundrums. *Family Court Review*. doi:10.1111/j.1744-1617.2009.01287.x.
5 Warshak, R.A. (2010). Family bridges: Using insights from social science to reconnect parents and alienated children. *Family Court Review*, 48, 48–80.
6 Heyes, C. (2018). Empathy is not in our genes. *Neuroscience and Biobehavioral Reviews*, 95, 499–507. doi:10.1016/j.neubiorev.2018.11.001.
7 Knafo, A., Zahn-Waxler, C., Van Hulle, C., Robinson, J.L. and Rhee, S.H. (2008). The developmental origins of a disposition towards empathy: Genetic and environmental contributions. *Emotion*, 8, 737–752. doi:10.1037/a0014179.
8 Abramson, L., Uzefovsky, F., Toccaceli, V. and Knafo-Noam, A. (2020). The genetic and environmental origins of emotional and cognitive empathy: Review and

meta-analyses of twin studies. *Neuroscience and Biobehavioral Reviews*, 114, 113–133. doi:10.1016/j.neubiorev.2020.03.023.

9 Asen, E. and Morris, E. (2020). *High-conflict parenting post-separation: The making and breaking of family ties*. Routledge.

10 Saputra, M.D., Joyoatmojo, S., Wardani, D.K. and Sangka, K.B. (2018). Developing critical thinking skills through the collaboration of jigsaw model with problem-based learning model. *International Journal of Instruction*, 12, 1077–1094.

11 Miller, W.R. and Rollnick, S. (1991). *Motivational interviewing: Preparing people to change addictive behaviour*. New York: Guildford Press.

12 Johannson, M., Damholdt, M.F., Zachariae, R., Lundorff, M., Farver-Vestergaard, I. and O'Connor, M. (2019). Psychological interventions for grief in adults: A systematic review and meta-analysis of randomised controlled trials. *Journal of Affective Disorders*, 253, 69–86. doi:10.1016/j.jad.2019.04.065.

13 Bisson, J.I. and Olff, M. (2021). Prevention and treatment of PTSD: The current evidence base. *European Journal of Psychotraumatology*, 12. doi:10.1080/20008198.2020.1824381.

14 Hofman, S.G., Asnaani, A., Vonk, I.J.J., Sawyer, A.T. and Fang, A. (2012). The efficacy of cognitive behavioural therapy: A review of the meta-analyses. *Cognitive Therapy and Research*, 36, 427–440.

15 Carr, A. (2008). The effectiveness of family therapy and systemic interventions for child-focused problems. *Journal of Family Therapy*, 31, 3–45. doi:10.1111/j.1467-6427.2008.00451.x.

16 Carr, A. (2008). The effectiveness of family therapy and systemic interventions for adult-focused problems. *Journal of Family Therapy*, 31, 46–74.

17 Linehan, M.M. (2015). *DBT skills training manual* (2nd edition). New York: The Guilford Press.

18 Gilbert, P. (2010). *Compassion focused therapy*. Oxon: Routledge.

19 Craig, C., Hiskey, S. and Spector, A. (2020). Compassion focused therapy: A systematic review of its effectiveness and acceptability in clinical populations. *Expert Review of Neurotherapeutics*, 20. doi:10.1080/14737175.2020.1746184.

20 Leaviss, J. and Uttley, L. (2015). Psychotherapeutic benefits of compassion-focused therapy: An early systematic review. *Psychological Medicine*, 45, 927–945. doi:10.1017/S0033291714002141.

21 Thomason, S. and Moghaddam, N. (2020). Compassion focused therapies for self-esteem: A systematic review and meta-analysis. *Psychology and Psychotherapy*. doi:10.1111/papt.12319.

22 Ben-Ami, N. and Baker, A.J.L. (2012). The long-term correlates of childhood exposure to parental alienation on adult self-sufficiency and well-being. *The American Journal of Family Therapy*, 40, 169–283.

23 Hayes, S.C., Strosahl, K.D. and Wilson, K.G. (1999). *Acceptance and commitment therapy: An experimental approach to behavior change*. New York: The Guilford Press.

24 Gloster, A.T., Walder, N., Levin, M.E., Twohig, M.P. and Karekla, M. (2020). The empirical status of acceptance and commitment therapy: A review of meta-analyses. *Journal of Contextual Behavioral Science*, 18, 181–192. doi:10.1016/j.jcbs.2020.09.009.

25 Byrne, G., Ní Ghráda, A., O'Mahony, T. and Brennan, E. (2020). A systematic review of the use of acceptance and commitment therapy in supporting parents. *Psychology and Psychotherapy*, 94, 378–407. doi:10.1111/papt.12282.

26 Keng, S.L., Smoski, M.J. and Robins, C.J. (2011). Effects of mindfulness on psychological health: A review of empirical studies. *Clinical Psychology Review*, 31, 1041–1056. doi:10.1016/j.cpr.2011.04.006.

27 Schumann, K. and Walton, G.M. (2021). Rehumanizing the self after victimization: The roles of forgiveness versus revenge. *Journal of Personality and Social Psychology*. doi:10.1037/pspi0000367.

28 de la Fuente-Anuncibay, R., González-Barbadillo, A., Ortega-Sánchez, D., Ordóñez-Camblor, N. and Pizarro-Ruiz, J.P. (2021). Anger rumination and mindfulness: Mediating effects on forgiveness. *International Journal of Environmental Research and Public Health*, 18, 2668. doi:10.3390/ijerph18052668.

29 Picard, L., Cousin, S., Guillery-Girard, B., Eustache, F. and Piolino, P. (2012). How do the different components of episodic memory develop? Role of executive functions and short-term feature-binding abilities. *Child Development*, 83, 1037–1050.

Chapter 12

What did we learn?

Introduction

Parental alienation is typically seen in the family courts, although it may also occur outside of this arena. It is a situation whereby an alienating parent manipulates a child such that they no longer wish to have a relationship with their other, targeted parent. Often the child had a positive relationship with the targeted parent before the separation. PA often involves allegations by the alienating parent of inappropriate behaviour on the part of the targeted parent. The inappropriate behaviour described can involve verbal, physical and/or sexual abuse. Often the child repeats what the alienating parent is saying and sometimes uses similar or adult language. In severely alienated families, the child might not have had contact with the targeted parent for many months or years, and uninformed experts can be concerned about recommending contact between a targeted parent and their child if there is a risk of abuse occurring. Therefore, the safest option is often to maintain the status quo and stop all contact with the targeted parent. This means that at times an innocent targeted parent loses contact with their child. In the meantime, a child does not see their targeted parent or their extended family, and they are left to believe that the targeted individuals pose a threat to them and sometimes that they do not care about them.

There is variability in the number and nature of allegations that are made, although typically a similar range of behaviours are present that have been described by many researchers across the globe (1–4). PA is on a continuum from mild to moderate to severe, and researchers have found that typically those families who have mildly alienating behaviour will progress to severely alienating if no intervention takes place (5). Examining a family situation and predicting the likelihood of abuse occurring is an important aspect of the court expert's work. It is also critical that the child, the alienating parent and the targeted parent are all listened to and that their information is considered in the context of their history. Professionals have to remain flexible and try to ensure that they do not misinterpret or misrepresent anything said by the parties involved, which can present a challenge in itself, given that a high level of emotion is often observed. Therefore, appropriate assessment and knowledge about the issues that are likely to occur is critical for anyone becoming involved with PA cases.

DOI: 10.4324/9781003156147-12

There have been significant efforts to try to study PA and consider the issues that are raised (1–6). Although some methodological issues have been raised about some of the studies, the contribution made to the existing body of knowledge is recognised (7). Due to the complexity of the cases, it is difficult to identify and measure the problems inherent in PA and compare groups. However, there is a shift towards trying to use more rigorous methodologies from a number of research groups (8–9).

Important outcomes that have been established are (a) when children are moved to the care of the targeted parent, they almost always appear to resolve the issues they have with them; (b) if children are left in the care of the alienating parent, the relationship with the targeted parent typically ends; and (c) alienation is not a gender issue; fathers and mothers are both capable of alienation (6, 9–11). Another critical piece of research found that adult children who felt they had been alienated from one parent later regretted this and experienced shame and guilt for the way they had treated their targeted parent (1). There are many reasons for establishing interventions and helping families involved in PA find a resolution.

Why the issues around parental alienation are so important

Recent studies into the changes in society over the past decade indicate that marriage and family are stable and likely to remain part of our culture (12), and we know that children of separated parents are happiest if they are supported to continue their relationships with their family. Family means different things to people, and sometimes close friendships can feel like family. The point is that if children feel family members do not care about them, then this is not good for their self-esteem and emotional welfare, and in addition, they miss out on all the possible benefits of engaging with the other part of their family. Also, if a child is caught in family disputes, then this can be destructive and harmful. From the parent's perspective, we know that they also experience better life satisfaction if the children split their time between both parents' homes. The benefits of positive decoupling and adjustment are significant.

Identification of parental alienation

Mild cases of PA will rarely reach court and might resolve without any intervention once the parents involved have adjusted to their new situation, whereas moderate and severe cases of PA will often end up in the family courts. Those who write extensively about PA note that some who argue against the use of the term believe it is used as a distraction in court by those who have been abusive and want to avoid any responsibility for a child's decision not to have contact with them (13). This is not consistent with the reports of many experts, who have assessed families where PA is an issue and found it to be present, and it also does not explain situations when people admit alienating behaviours. In addition, the problems of PA are described by many court experts across the globe, who are independent of each other and are trying to find answers to the difficulties seen.

Some authors claim that an allegation of PA is used inappropriately at times to minimise the experiences of women who have been physically mistreated by their ex-partners (14). It has been reported that an allegation of parental alienation increases the likelihood that woman and children will be doubted in the Family Court. It is proposed that an allegation is more likely if a resident mother (there is no reference to resident fathers) indicates that she feels her children may not be safe in the care of her ex-partner. It is believed that as a result, children are forced to have contact with abusive ex-partners. A number of issues are raised by this claim, for example whether children should have contact with abusive ex-partners, particularly if there is no evidence of violence or abuse other than one parent's allegations and if there is no history of the parent being abusive to the child.

There is a growing interest in and recognition of the impact of PA on children, and it is increasingly being recognised as a form of domestic violence. However, identifying PA is not an effort to undermine adults who have genuine concerns about their ex-partner or distract from these. In PA, when professionals are unsure whether violence against a child has occurred, then contact with the targeted parent is supervised, until or if professionals are content that the child is safe.

Interventions

Family therapy has been used with some success for the mild and some moderate cases; however, the efficacy in severe cases is poor. Attempts to try to bring about change whilst the child is in the care of the alienating parent have not been hugely successful. Children are sometimes removed to the care of the targeted parent, and modified family therapy can be introduced to try to help families establish a new 'normal' after the child has been moved. There have been positive outcome studies when these programmes have been introduced (10).

Other approaches have been attempted with some success, and despite the poor outcomes for interventions whilst the child remains in the care of the alienating parent, it is difficult for any professional person to suggest removal of a child from their preferred parent. Recently some attempts have been made to try to reduce the impact and permanence of any separation between the alienating/preferred parent and child by offering temporary removal of the child and supervised contact with the alienating parent whilst they have an opportunity to engage with therapeutic intervention tailored to their needs. In the meantime, the child resides with the targeted parent and/or their family. This offers an opportunity to the alienating parent to work towards a shared-care arrangement and at the same time enables the targeted parent and child to work towards establishing a relationship again.

The needs of the family differ depending on the nature of their difficulties, and there are thousands of publications that provide evidence for the use of a range of therapies for specific difficulties and mental health problems. Focus on the current interventions used in clinical practice can be applied to some of the problems seen in PA, although it requires an individual approach for each case. The benefit of this approach means that the individuals involved will have access to the recommended and evidence-based interventions if they need them. It might be the case that intervention only results in helping an alienating parent improve their emotional functioning after their child is removed from their care, rather than working towards a shared-care arrangement. This will occur if the alienating parent continues not to want to engage in a shared parenting arrangement. However, the alienating parent also has an opportunity to reflect on the reasons for their decision to alienate their child and to engage in any intervention offered to try to bring about change. Not all alienating parents are able to do this.

Can parents be helped not to alienate their children?

It could be argued that as the focus is to meet the needs of the child, then whichever parent can best support the child's need to have a relationship with both parents and extended family should be the resident parent.

Parenting classes and education during the early stages of separation can help prevent or ameliorate mild alienation, but most of the parents who care enough about their children to find out about the consequences of their child not having a relationship with their other parent are unlikely to become alienating parents. In my experience alienating parents do not respond to advice that they are harming their child.

The role of professionals

It has been suggested that experts could be relied on in PA cases; however, it is important that they are educated about PA and also about domestic violence or intimate partner violence (IPV) (14). It is really important that the expert can identify when a situation appears to be PA and when there are other reasons for the presentation (13). There are concerns about whether if PA is identified the targeted parent is considered the more reliable parent, since the alienating parent might hold a view that is not consistent with the findings of the expert. This and the many issues associated with correct identification highlight the importance for professionals involved to be extremely vigilant and ensure the term is not abused (13).

Final word

There is a significant literature that acknowledges the presence of PA, and many writers have also criticised the concept. What the literature has in common is a shared belief in meeting the best interests of the child, and family violence is not condoned by anyone. The differences between the various views have been argued in this text and in others. A positive approach would involve accepting parental alienation as a particular form of family violence (8), as serious as physical and other emotional and psychological violence, but with the understanding that not all allegations of violence (including PA) are true and knowing that each case needs to be considered on its own merits.

There are allegations of confirmation bias in some documents, which undermines the knowledge of professionals involved, since it suggests that legal and health and social care professionals are jumping to conclusions and trying to confirm PA (15). It is of course paramount to the assessment that experts are independent and knowledgeable, and professionals need to understand PA so that they can identify when it is alleged but does not exist (13).

It is generally understood that some parents inappropriately manipulate their children to cause deterioration to their relationship with the other parent and that this presents a significant problem for families and the courts. Court experts and other professionals involved are highly sensitive to the issues associated with allegations of abusive behaviours. No one wants to be responsible for a child having to spend time with an abusive parent; however, at the same time, false allegations mean that innocent parents lose contact with their child. With the best interests of the child at the core of every decision, professionals are focused on ensuring that recommendations made are safe and helpful, although even after considerable investigation it is not always possible to say with certainty that a child will be safe in the care of either parent.

Parental alienation as a concept has been established, and whilst appropriate interventions and associated recommendations for families as a group might remain elusive, it is clear that PA occurs, it is harmful and that it needs to be addressed.

References

1 Baker, A.J.L. (2005). The long-term effects of parental alienation on adult children: A qualitative research study. *American Journal of Family Therapy*, 33, 289–302. doi:10.1080/01926180590962129.

2 Harman, J.J., Bernet, W. and Harman, J. (2019). Parental alienation: The blossoming of a field of study. *Current Directions in Psychological Science*, 28. doi:10.1177/0963721419827271.

3 Warshak, R.A. (2010). Family bridges: Using insights from social science to reconnect parents and alienated children. *Family Court Review*, 48, 48–80. doi:10.1111./j.1744-1617.2009.01288.x.

4 Haines, J., Matthewson, M. and Turnbull, M. (2020). *Understanding and managing parental alienation: A guide to assessment and intervention*. Oxon: Routledge.

5 Roma, P., Marchetti, D., Mazza, C., Burla, F. and Verrocchio, M.C. (2020). MMPI-2 profiles of mothers engaged in parental alienation. *Journal of Family Issues*, 1–10. doi:10.1177/0192513X20918393.

6 Ben-Ami, N. and Baker, A.J.L. (2012). The long-term correlates of childhood exposure to parental alienation on adult self-sufficiency and well-being. *The American Journal of Family Therapy*, 40, 169–283.

7   Saini, M., Johnston, J.R., Fidler, B.J. and Bala, N. (2016). Empirical studies of aliena-
    tion. In L. Drozd, M. Saini and N. Oleson (Eds.), *Parenting plan evaluations: Applied
    research for the family court* (pp. 374–430). Oxford University Press. doi:10.1093/
    med:psych/9780199396580.003.0013.
8   Harman, J.J., Kruk, E. and Hines, D. (2018). Parental alienating behaviours: An unac-
    knowledged form of family violence. *Psychological Bulletin*, 144, 1275–1299.
9   Templer, K., Matthewson, M., Haines, J. and Cox, G. (2016). Recommendations for
    best practice in response to parental alienation: Findings from a systematic review.
    Journal of Family Therapy, 39, 103–122. doi:10.1111/1467-6427.12137.
10 Warshak, R.A. (2015). Parental alienation: Overview, management, intervention and
    practice tips. *Journal of the American Academy of Matrimonial Lawyers*, 28, 181–248.
11 Harman, J.J., Biringen, Z., Ratajck, E.M., Outland, P.L. and Kraus, A. (2016). Parents
    behaving badly: Gender biases in the perception of parental alienation. *Journal of
    Family Psychology*, 30, 866–874. doi:10.1037/fam0000232.
12 Kelly Raley, R. and Sweeney, M.M. (2020). Divorce, re-partnering and stepfami-
    lies: A decade in review. *Journal of Marriage and Family*, 82, 81–89. doi:10.1111/
    jomf.12651.
13 Warshak, R.A. (2019). When evaluators get it wrong: False positive IDs and parental
    alienation. *Psychology, Public Policy and Law*, 26, 54–68. doi:10.1037/law0000216.
14 Mackenzie, D., Herbert, R. and Robertson, N. (2020). 'It's not OK', but 'it' never hap-
    pened: Parental alienation accusations undermine children's safety in the New Zealand
    family court. *Journal of Social Welfare and Family Law*, 42, 106–117. doi:10.1080/
    09649069.2020.1701942.
15 Sheehy, E. and Boyd, S.B. (2020). Penalizing women's fear: Intimate partner violence
    and parental alienation in Canadian child custody cases. *Journal of Social Welfare and
    Family Law*, 42, 80–91. doi:10.1080/09649069.2020.1701940.

Index

Page numbers in **bold** indicate a table on the corresponding page.